PLAB 2
Course Book

Companion Volume

Highway to PLAB 2 :
Objective Structured Clinical Examination

This book is designed to be used with the NHS Recruits PLAB 2
Course and Tutorials. Extensive manikin practice is done at the
course along with communication skills stations.

visit
www.nhsrecruits.com
for PLAB 2 Course and Clinical Attachment

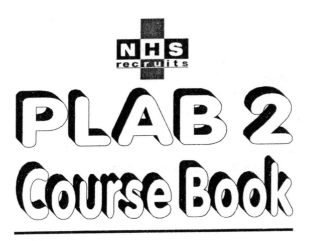

PLAB 2
Course Book

Zakir H Patel
Tauseef Azim
Arif Dasu

CBS

CBS PUBLISHERS & DISTRIBUTORS
NEW DELHI • BANGALORE

NHS Recruits
PLAB 2 Course Book

First Edition : 2004
　　Reprint : 2005

Copyright © 2004, Authors and Publishers

ISBN : 81-239-1048-7

Production Director : Vinod K. Jain

Published by :
Satish Kumar Jain for CBS Publishers & Distributors,
4596/1-A, 11 Darya Ganj, New Delhi - 110 002 (India)
E-mail : cbspubs@del3.vsnl.net.in
Website : http://www.cbspd.com

Branch Office :
Seema House, 2975, 17th Cross, K.R. Road,
Bansankari 2nd Stage, Bangalore - 560070
Fax : 080-6771680 • E-mail : cbsbng@vsnl.net

Printed at :
Asia Printograph, Shahdara, Delhi - 110032 (India)

PLAB Examination

It consists of 14 stations. Each lasts 5 minutes. You will have a test station that does not count towards your final mark. You will be graded A–excellent, B–good, C–adequate, D–fail and E–severe fail. To pass PLAB 2, a candidate must get a minimum of grade C for ten of the stations and must not have received a grade E for more than one station.

It is not impossible to pass. Be **sensible** and be **polite** in the examination. If you do not know an answer for something, do not say something silly. Tell the examiner that you will ask your senior or look it up in a book.

Be calm, you will not be expected to know everything.

Work as a **group** when training. Learn from each other. It will also improve your communication skills.

Attend a **course** so that you can brush up on communication and manikin skills.

Organise a **clinical attachment** for four–six weeks.

RECOMMENDED BOOKLIST

Surgery

• *An Introduction to the Symptoms and Signs of Surgical Disease,* Norman, K. MD FRCS FRCP, Browse.

• *Surgical Finals: Passing the Clinical,* Gina Kuperberg, John Lumley.

Medicine

• *Core Clinical Skills for OSCEs in Medicine,* Tim Dornan, O'Neill.

• *Oxford Handbook of Clinical Medicine,* J.M. Longmore, Murray Longmore, Ian Wilkinson, Estee Torok.

• *Oxford Handbook of Clinical Specialties,* J.A.B. Collier, J.M. Longmore.

• *Clinical Medicine 5/e,* Parveen Kumar & Michael Clark, WB Saunders, London.

Paediatrics

• *Illustrated Textbook of Paediatrics,* Tom, MB BChir FRCP Lissauer, Graham, MD FRCPP, Clayden.

PLAB OSCEs

• *PLAB 2: 100 Objective Structured Clinical Examinations,* Dr Una Coales MD FRCS FRCSO DRCOG DFFP.

• *The Complete PLAB: OSCEs,* M Afzal Mir, Srinivasan Madhusudan, Anne E. Freeman.

Obstetrics and Gynaecology

• *Essential Obstetrics and Gynaecology,* E.Malcolm Symonds.

Psychiatry

• *Psychiatry in Medical Practice, 2/e,* D. Goldberg.

Examination Skills

• *Macleods Clinical Examination,* J F Munro, I W Campbell.

*NHS notes have most of the information needed.

Acknowledgements

I would like to thank first of all God who gave me the guidance and knowledge to make this possible, my parents for making me what I am, my wife and children for giving me inspiration, and Tauseef for all his encouragement and work.

Zakir H Patel

plab@nhsrecruits.com.

Contents

EMERGENCIES   *1*

Basic Life Support *1*
  Adult *1*
  Paediatric *3*
Venepuncture *5*
Cannulation *6*
Catheterization *8*
  Male *8*
  Female *9*
Wounds *10*
Suturing *11*

MEDICINE   *13*

CVS Examination *13*
Blood Pressure Monitoring *17*
Respiratory Examination *19*
Inhaler Use *23*
Peak Flow Meter *24*
Spacer *26*
Neurological Examination *27*
Diabetic Lower Limb Examination *32*
Thyroid Examination *34*
Ophthalmoscopy *37*
Ear Examination: Otoscopy *40*
Chest Pain and MI Advice *42*
Asthma *47*
Panic Attacks and Palpitations *49*
TIA or Stroke *51*
Headache *53*
Epilepsy *59*

Weightloss *63*
Analgesia *65*
Diabetic Ketoacidosis Management *67*
Fever *69*
Joints *71*
DVT/PE *73*
Postmortems/Death Certificate *75*

COMMUNICATION 78

History Taking *78*
Phoning for Advice *80*
Consent *83*
In Summary *86*
Breaking Bad News *90*

SURGERY 96

Abdominal Pain *96*
PR Bleeding *98*
Haematuria *99*
Scaphoid *101*
Needlestick Injury *102*
Abdominal Examination *103*
Testicular Examination *105*
Rectal Examination *107*
Arterial System *109*
Venous System *111*
Spine Examination *113*
  Cervical *113*
  Thoracic *115*
  Lumbar *116*
Hand Examination *119*
Shoulder Examination *121*
Hip Examination *122*
Knee Examination *124*

OBSTETRICS AND GYNAECOLOGY　　　*127*

History Taking　*128*
HRT　*129*
Contraception Advice　*131*
Ectopics　*133*
　Counselling　*135*
Sterilization　*137*
Vasectomy　*139*
Cervical Smears　*141*
STD　*143*
Termination of Pregnancy　*145*
Pre-Eclampsia　*147*
Post-Natal Depression　*149*
Amenorrhoea　*151*
Hyperemesis　*152*
Cervical Smear Results　*153*
Bimanual/Speculum Examination　*154*
Breast Examination　*158*

PAEDIATRICS　　　*160*

Cases　*160*
Talking to Mother on the Phone　*161*
?Meningitis　*163*
Advice about Diarrhoea　*165*
Stillborn baby　*166*
Colic　*168*
Crying Baby　*171*
Polydipsia　*172*
Child has Asthma　*173*
Febrile Convulsion　*175*
Nocturnal Enuresis　*176*
Non-Accidental Injury　*177*
Talking to Parents　*178*

PSYCHIATRY   *179*

History Taking *179*
Mental State Examination *181*
Mini Mental State *184*
Alcohol *187*
Drug Abuse *190*
Paracetamol Overdose *192*
Depression *195*
Suicide *196*

EMERGENCIES

BASIC LIFE SUPPORT

In Summary:

ADULTS

Scenario: 'Some elderly gentleman has collapsed in front of you in the supermarket or called to collapsed adult on ward'

1. Approach area – Make sure safe, i.e. no risk of electrocution, motor cars, etc.
2. "Are you all right?
3. Shout 'HELP'
4. Open airway and clear it of obstruction
5. Check breathing for 10 secs – LOOK, LISTEN, FEEL
6. If no response – CRASH CALL – go yourself if on own*
    If response – RECOVERY POSITION
7. On returning 2 rescue breaths (assuming no breathing) – up to five attempts
8. Check carotid pulse for 10 secs
9. 15 × sternal compression (assuming no pulse) – 2 fingers above base of sternum. Rate of 100, using two hands and pressing 4–5 cm.

10. Repeat from 7
11. Reassess every minute

ONCE DEFIB ARRIVES – USE IT. AS THIS IS WHAT WILL SAVE LIFE

- Adults who are victims of TRAUMA or DROWNING should have resuscitation for 1 minute before going for help if on own. This is because these groups are more likely to be suffering from hypoxia (respiratory cause).

PAEDIATRIC LIFE SUPPORT

More likely due to respiratory cause than cardiac

Exactly same as above but some slight changes.

INFANT < 1yr

1. Safe approach
2. 'Are you all right?'
3. Open airway (<12 months head in neutral position and if >12 months 'sniffing morning air' position)
4. Look inside mouth for FB
5. LOOK, LISTEN, FEEL
6. 2 rescue breaths over 1.5–2 secs
7. Check pulse (brachial) for 10 secs
8. CPR (5 chest compressions) – 100 min using two fingers and a ratio of 5:1. Also, do cardiac compressions if pulse <60.
9. Repeat from point 6 for 1 minute.
10. After 1 minute of CPR call ambulance. If on own go yourself.
11. When returning restart from beginning.
    - Infants (<12 months) – use 2 fingers one finger below nipple line
    - <4 years – use 1 hand one finger above xiphisternum
    - <12 years – use 1–2 hands two fingers above xiphisternum

NB: Do one minute before calling for help if you are on your own.

CHILD 1–8 years

1. Safe approach
2. 'Are you all right?'
3. Open airway (<12 months head in neutral pos. and if >12 months 'sniffing morning air' position).
4. Look inside mouth for FB
5. LOOK, LISTEN, FEEL
6. 2 rescue breaths over 1.5–2 secs. Again five attempts max.
7. Check pulse (carotid) for 10 secs.
8. CPR (5 chest compressions) – 100 min using one hand and one finger above base of sternum and a ratio of 5:1. Also, do cardiac compressions if pulse <60.
9. Repeat from point 6 for 1 minute.
10. After 1 minute of CPR call ambulance (roughly 12 cycles). If on own, go yourself.
11. When returning, restart from beginning.

Remember **INTRAOSSEUS INFUSION**

Useful Calculations

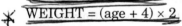

WEIGHT = (age + 4) × 2

E.T. TUBE size = (Age/4) + 4

Joules for DEFIB. = (2 × kg) J, (2 × kg) J and (4 × kg) J

Visit: www.resus.org.uk

* Protocols + Defibrillation – See Booklet or Course

VENEPUNCTURE

Greet patient and introduce yourself. Explain procedure to patient and what taking blood for.

1. Get permission and check patient name and d.o.b. on name band.
2. Check your equipment, i.e. needle, appropriate bottles, alcowipe, cotton, sharps bin, plaster, gloves and tourniquet.
3. Wear gloves (do not have to be sterile).
4. Palpate to feel vein.
5. Wipe with alcowipe. Make sure you do not touch again.
6. Pierce through skin (NB: pointed bit should pierce first).
7. Pull syringe back and allow blood to drain.
8. Once full, remove blood bottle, leave needle in.
9. Fill second bottle, if needed.
10. Remove tourniquet.
11. Place cotton wool on pierced area and remove needle.
12. Throw needle in sharps bin.
13. "Thank you". If fail, apologise and ask to try elsewhere.
14. Label and fill form out.

CANNULATION (VENFLON)

Greet patient and introduce yourself. Explain procedure to patient and why inserting cannula, i.e. to give medicines.

1. Get permission and check patient name and d.o.b. on name band.
2. Check your equipment, i.e. cannula, alcowipe, cotton, sharps bin, plaster, gloves and tourniquet.
3. Wear gloves (do not have to be sterile).
4. Palpate to feel vein.
5. Wipe with alcowipe. Make sure you don't touch again.
6. Pierce needle through skin slightly more than that for taking blood.
7. Once in vein, get flashback, i.e. blood in cannula.
8. Start pushing in mid-plastic region until end fairly near the pierced point.
9. Now as well as pushing plastic bit in, start withdrawing needle nearly pulled out.
10. Take tourniquet off.
11. Once tourniquet off, put finger on vein (upstream).
12. Discard needle in sharps bin.
13. Attach cap to cannula.
14. Stick cannula down.

15. Flush with normal saline.
16. "Thank you".

NB: If fail, don't worry. Apologise to patient and ask to try again. If fail after three attempts, ask a colleague to have ago.

NB: In the exam manikins you may not get a **flashback**. This is usually not because you have not hit the vein but because the manikins are faulty. If this happens to you DON'T PANIC – tell the examiner that you are not getting a flashback and in a real patient you would restart, however, clarify that 'is this because of the manikins here.' He will probably tell you to continue.

CATHETERISATION

MALE CATHETERISATION

Greet patient and introduce yourself.

Explain what you intend to do and why, i.e. get verbal consent.

Collect all equipment

1. Wash hands.
2. Wear gloves.
3. Place a sterile towel around penis.
4. Retract foreskin and clean glans area. NB: Clean penis area first if it was dirty.
5. Retract penis backward and hold.
6. Pour in urethra 10–15 ml of sterile anaesthetic and lubrication gel.
7. Wait 4–5 minutes.
8. Push catheter in gently. Once get to external urethral sphincter you get some resistance and so push pass it. Do not force. To make passing past sphincter easier, ask patient to 'cough' or 'try to pass water'.
9. Once in, urine passes.
10. Blow up balloon using 10 ml water.
11. Pull back catheter until balloon holds at tip of bladder.
12. Attach bag.

FEMALE CATHETERIASTION

Greet patient and introduce yourself.

Explain what you intend to do and why, i.e. get verbal consent.

Collect all equipment

1. Wash hands.
2. Wear gloves.
3. Place a sterile towel around genitalia.
4. Clean area on both sides of labia majora.
5. Put two fingers into labia majora area to raise it.
6. Put catheter through urethra (top hole). Hold catheter facing upwards – makes it easier.
7. Once get urine, you are in bladder (NB: Women do not have external urethral sphincter so there is no resistance).
8. Blow up balloon using 10 ml water.
9. Attach bag.

WOUNDS

- Site
- Size
- Shape
- Sharp = Incision/
- Blunt =Laceration
- Sterile (is it clean?)
- Structures (underlying nerves, tendons, vessels affected)
- Always X-ray if suspect foreign body
- TETANUS (lasts 10 yrs)
- You can close with sutures, steristrips, glue, etc.

SUTURING

- Introduce.
- Explain.
- Establish that there is full range of movement and there is no neurovascular compromise or tendon injury.
- Inform the patient to lie in supine position.
- Requirements
  - A good source of light.
  - Suturing materials.
  - LA
  - Syringe.
- Sterilze
- Anaesthetize with 10 ml Lignocaine infiltration
- Wait (5–10 minutes).
- Tell the patient that she will feel pressure but not pain.
- Apply suture over the wound.
- Dispose
  - Sharps   - sharp bin
  - Clinical waste   - yellow bin
  - Paper   - black bin
  - Glass   - orange bin
- Inform the patient that the sutures will need to be removed in a week's time.
- Inform the patient that if he develops temperature, wound breakdown, or wound discharge, he should return to the casualty or see his GP soon.

- Give painkillers.
- Consider immunization and vaccination against tetanus if indicated
- Say 'Thanks'.
- Antiseptic solutions as hydrogen peroxide or betadine.

MEDICINE

CARDIOVASCULAR EXAMINATION

When examining patient always

- **Introduce**
- **Be polite**
- **Ask patient's permission**
- **Tell patient before doing anything**
- **Ensure privacy**
- **Ask for a chaperone**
- **Look around patient's bed for any clues, e.g. GTN spray, inhalers, etc.**
- **Ask the patient "Are you comfortable?"**

1. Approach patient from RIGHT hand side.

2. Introduce and ask for permission "I am Dr ____. How are you today? Is it OK if I examine you? You will have to take your shirt/blouse off. Is that all right? Do you require a chaperone?"

3. Check hands. Look at **nails** properly. Feel surface of nails. Get nails at eye-level and look at sides. Look for **clubbing**. If you put two nails together, you should get a diamond

shape. Look for **splinter haemorrhages, capillary refill** (should be <3 secs). Are hands cold/sweaty?

4. Look at palms. Look at colour and look in creases. Look for cholesterol and nicotine staining.

5. Run thumb down the tendons on back of hand to feel for cholesterol deposits – tendon **xanthomata**. Feel for hardening of blood vessels due to cholesterol.

6. Feel radial pulse for 15 secs. Look at **rate/ rhythm,** i.e. 60/minute regular.

7. Compare pulse with other hand and look for radio-femoral delay. Tell patient that you are feeling for a pulse in the groin.

8. Ask patient if they have any shoulder pain. Then raise arm to 90°. Feel pulse and feel for water-hammer pulse (aortic regurgurgitation).

9. Feel brachial pulse with thumb. It is medial to biceps tendon. Here check for **volume and character**.

10. Say "I would like to check your BP."

11. Do jugular venous pressure (**JVP**). Get patient to relax on bed at 45°. Ask patient to look to the left. Hopefully, you should be able to see a pulsation. Measure the vertical height of the pulsation from the sternal angle. NB: you will actually see two pulsations (i.e. a and c wave of JVP.)

12. Feel carotid pulse.

13. Check eyes. Pull bottom eyelids down and see if red, i.e. not anaemic. Check around cornea for **corneal arcus**. Check conjunctiva is not yellow – jaundiced. Check below eyes for cholesterol deposits, i.e. **xanthalasma**.

14. Tongue – ask to pull tongue out and make sure no central cyanosis. Do this by asking the patient to raise tongue, i.e. put tip of tongue on upper teeth.

15. Chest – take a step back and look at chest. Look for any scars, abnormal breathing pattern, deformities, pulsations, etc.

16. Place whole hand under the left nipple and palpate to feel apex. Then localize with two and then one finger. Once found apex, count ribs, etc. to localize exact position, e.g. 5th intercostals space mid-clavicular line.

17. Put hand on nipple around apex. See if there is a heave, i.e. heel of hand should lift. This shows left ventricular hypertrophy. Next put hand on pulmonary and aortic valve region and feel for thrills.

18. Auscultate the valves. First do apex with diaphragm (big part of stethoscope) and then using bell. When listening for at apex feel pulse. Then feel rest of valves using diaphragm.

NB: When doing pulmonary valve, ask patient to hold breath on inspiration (increases intensity of sound). Once done, ask patient to continue breathing normally.

19. Using bell auscultate carotid. Ask patient to hold breath while listening for thrill, etc. maximum length of time for holding breath <5 secs.

20. Ask patient to lean forwards and breath in and then hold breath on expiration. Listen for aortic regurgitation (with diaphragm).

21. Ask patient to sit forwards. Percuss back.

22. Auscultate back.

23. Check for sacral oedema on back.

24. Check ankle oedema.

25. Feel liver for hepatomegaly, pulsations, aneurysm, enlarged kidneys.

26. Check peripheral pulses.

27. In the end tell examiner that you would like to check BP, fundoscopy, urine, peripheral pulses and obs chart.

28. Thank the patient for their cooperation.

BLOOD PRESSURE MONITORING

Very common scenario. Explain to the patient by saying, "I would like to check your blood pressure. I will be putting this cuff around your arm and it will go tight. It will feel uncomfortable but not painful. You may feel tingling in your hands – tell me if you do please."

1. Check the sphygmomanometer is working and set to zero.
2. Choose an appropriate-sized cuff.
3. Wrap cuff around arm with bladder over brachial artery.
4. Support arm at heart level.
5. Inflate cuff while palpating brachial artery and calculate systolic pressure by palpation.
6. Deflate cuff back to zero.
7. Inflate cuff again going 20–30 mmHg over the palpated systolic pressure.
8. Record systolic and diastolic pressure to the nearest 2 mmHg and record result with units (mmHg). Note use Korotkov sound 4.
9. Now tell the patient "I would like to recheck your blood pressure while you are standing."
10. Ask the patient to stand up with cuff deflated still around arm. Ask patient "Are you feeling dizzy?" If the patient feels dizzy, ask him/her to sit the down/lie down and ask for help.

11. Recheck BP while standing. If there is a drop of 20 mm Hg which is sustained at 2 min then there is postural hypotension.

Raised BP is >160/90 mmHg. Diastolic between 90–99 mmHg is borderline – moderate hypertension and you would treat this if patient had other risk factors, e.g. diabetes, smoker, etc.

RESPIRATORY EXAMINATION

1. Approach patient from RIGHT hand side
2. Introduce and ask for permission "I am Dr ____. How are you today? Is it OK if I examine you? You will have to take your shirt/blouse off – strip to waist, is that all right? Do you require a chaperone?"
3. Stand at the **end of the bed** and ask the patient to breath in and out. Look at the chest for colour, deformity– pigeon and funnel-shaped chest, symmetry, scars, etc.
4. Check hands. Look for:
   - Nicotine staining
   - Clubbing
   - Muscle wasting on hand
   - CO_2 retention flap. Ask patient to hold arms out straight – hand bent so that fingers are pointing upwards. Fingers should be spread out
   - Wrist pain – pulmonary osteoarthropathy
5. Check pulse. Get down to side of bed and watch chest movement at same time. Measure pulse for 15 secs and measure respiratory rate also for 15 secs. Normal rate 12–16/min.
6. Measure JVP. Can get raised JVP in pulmonary hypertension.
7. Check face. Check for anaemia and jaundice. Also, check for Horner's syndrome. Here get

a constricted pupil and no sweat on that side of the face. Check for ptosis.

8. Ask patient to open mouth and say 'ARRGH'. Using pen-torch check inside mouth for enlarged tonsils. Check underneath tongue for central cyanosis.

9. Ask patient to block one nostril and sniff. This is to check that nasal airways are not blocked.

10. Palpate trachea. Warn patient that s/he may feel uncomfortable. Use two fingers just above sternal notch for this.

11. Chest – **look** at chest for deformities, barrel chest, injuries, scars, etc.

12. Expansion – check chest expansion using thumbs.

13. **Percussion** – start by percussing apex of lungs. Move down. NB over clavicles you do not need to percuss on fingers, i.e. percuss directly onto clavicles. Continue to just below nipple line.

Find apex beat.

Also, feel for crepitus (surgical emphysema)

14. **Auscultate** – use the diaphragm. If you think there is any pathology, then use the bell. NB: when using the diaphragm you need to press hard enough to leave an impression but not too hard as to hurt the patient!

15. Vocal resonance – ask patient to say '99' and auscultate lung areas.

16. Check neck lymph nodes. Remember ant/post. triangle, submandibular and auricular glands.
17. Ask patient to sit forwards. Look at the back of the chest and spine. Do same to back, e.g. percuss, auscultate, etc.
18. Check for ankle oedema.
19. Ask examiner that you would like to check sputum, PFR (if relevant), temperature.
20. Thank the patient.

INHALER USE

"Hello Mrs Jones, my name is Dr ____. Is it OK if I teach you how to use the inhaler most effectively?"

"1. Check your inhaler is not finished or out of date. Most new inhalers have a counter and show the number of doses left.

2. Shake the inhaler.

3. Breathe out fully and place mouthpiece in mouth. Hold it firmly between the lips.

4. Now you need to take a deep breath in. At the same time as you start breathing in, press the top of the inhaler so that you get a dose of the drug. You should feel the drug at the back of your mouth, if taken correctly.

5. Hold your breath for 10 secs (easy way to do this is count 1 elephant, 2 elephant ... 10 elephant)."

6. Do this yourself so that patient understands.

7. Ask patient to do it in front of you.

8. Repeat same again if need further doses.

9. If using a steroid inhaler, ask patient to rinse mouth out afterwards to prevent thrush infection.

NB: There are different types of inhalers. In the exam you are most likely to get a metered dose inhaler (MDI). Technique to use this is as described above. The other types are 'easy-breath' no need to press the gas canister, just breathe in and the drug is delivered automatically. Turbohaler—just twist the inhaler clockwise to get a dose ready. Auto-haler—has a red lever that you need to lift first. Accuhaler—depress lever to activate.

PEAK FLOW METER

"Hello, Mrs Jones, my name is Dr _____. I would like to show you how to use a device called peak flow meter. It looks like this. We use it so that we can monitor your asthma and see if the treatment we are giving you is effective. It is very easy to use but needs some skill. Let me show you:

1. To be most accurate, it has to be used standing up if possible.
2. Take a deep breath in and then place the mouth piece in your mouth before exhaling. Make sure that you are not obstructing the markers on the peak flow meter with your fingers.
3. Now blow out as hard and fast as you can.
4. Look at the reading and write it down.
5. Repeat the procedure two more times. Record the best result in your book.
6. I would like you to do this twice a day. Once in morning and then at night.
7. Do you follow? (Do the procedure yourself once and then ask the patient: "Please show me how to do it now.")
8. If you have taken an extra inhaler dose just before testing or if you have a cold at the time please mark it in your diary so we can compare the results for those dates.
9. I will see you in 4 weeks time with the results. In the meantime if there is any problem you

can contact the asthma specialist nurse who can advise you.

10. Thank you. Any questions?"

SPACER

"Hello Sir, my name is Dr _____. Is it OK if I talk to you about a device called a spacer? It looks like this and it will help you get more of the inhaler drug into your lungs.

1. The spacer looks conical in shape. You need to put the two bits together like this.
2. This end is where the inhaler fits—like this.
3. The other end you place inside your mouth. This end has a valve so that it will only open when you breathe in.
4. Once you have assembled the spacer, shake your inhaler and insert it into the inhaler end of the space – like this.
5. Now breathe out slowly and then place the breathing side of the spacer into your mouth.
6. Press the inhaler once and breath in deeply.
7. Hold your breath for 10 secs.
8. To clean spacer just use water and allow to dry in air. Do it once a week."
9. Do the procedure yourself and demonstrate to the patient, then ask patient to repeat.

NEUROLOGICAL EXAMINATION

You may be asked to examine cranial nerves or asked to examine the lower limb, in which case you would have to check neurology and vascular joints. If they ask for just neurological examination then start with cranial nerves and then move to peripheral nervous examination.

Cranial Nerves

I
- "Can you smell normally?" There are some special smells you could use but not for the examination.

II
- Visual acuity (Snellen chart).
  Visual fields – do one eye at a time.
  Waving finger method in periphery is fine.
- Reflexes (direct and consensual).
  Accommodation (look at object in distance and then held close).
  Fundoscopy.

III,IV, VI – Eye movements.
- Look for squint and nystagmus.
- Move sideways and then up and down. Look for nystagmus (which direction).
- If diplopia ask which direction it is in and which eye.

V
- Check sensation in the three regions.
- Motor function – muscles of mastication. Look for wasting. Ask patient to bite or

open mouth against resistance. Also, check jaw jerk – place your thumb over mandible, tap with tendon hammer on thumb. Patient's jaw will close (bite) with normal reflex.

VII • Look for symmetry of facial muscles. Raise eyebrows, wrinkle forehead, close eyes and prevent opening. Show teeth and blow. For sensory part can do Schirmer's test or taste in anterior two-thirds of tongue .

• Mention corneal reflex – will not be asked to do.

VIII • Check hearing – whisper numbers in patient's ear – ask to repeat.

• Rinnes test – place tuning fork on mastoid process and then to ear. Ask "which is louder?" If louder on mastoid then conduction defect.

• Weber test – put tuning fork in mid of forehead. Ask "which side can you hear it?" Will hear on side of conductive deafness. Have a look at ears with otoscope. May want to do Hallpike's if suspect BPPV.

IX/X • Assess patient's speech.

• Ask patient to say 'aargh' watch palate move symmetrically.

• You will not have to do 'gag' but just mention that you would like to do.

XI • Look for weakness on trapezius or sterno-clomastoid.

• Ask patient to shrug shoulders against resistance. To test left sternomastoid, ask patient to look to the right while you resist this movement.

XII • Ask patient to protrude tongue in and out. Look for fasciculation's. Ask patient to move tongue side to side. Push against cheek and check power.

Peripheral Nervous System —

Easiest way to do this is to split examination into:

- Look for wasting, fasciculation's, hypertrophy.
- Tone – increased (upper motor neurone lesion) or decreased (lower motor prob.), passively flex knee, etc. and check for clonus.
- Power – check all movements, e.g. elbow flex/ extend. MRC Grades 0=none, 1=flicker, 2=cannot lift against gravity, 3=can lift against gravity, 4=overcomes resistance, 5=normal.
- Reflexes – biceps (C5/C6), triceps (C6/C7), supinator (C5 tap onto your thumb), knee (L3/ L4) and ankle (S1).
- Sensation: Check on patients sternum first, i.e. put cotton wool on sternum and say 'remember this sensation.' Then put cotton wool on area to be tested, e.g. limb and say 'is this the same as on your chest?' If yes, normal. Map out dermatomes. Test touch (cotton wool), sharp pain (disposable pin), heat, vibration (start with distal joints first, if sensation present in distal joint then not necessary to check peripheral ones. Mention to examiner that as distal sensation is normal, you presume so will be the proximal.

- Plantar reflex
- Gait

1. Introduce yourself and ask patient to undress to underwear if checking whole body. Ensure privacy and get chaperone. Ask patient to Relax.

2. Check for muscle wasting on arms, legs, etc. compare one side to other.

3. Check tone of upper limb, i.e. move elbow, wrist and fingers.

4. Ask the patient to flex shoulders, i.e. hold shoulders up and push from top of arms downwards. Then do same but push upwards this time.

5. Ask the patient to flex elbows and you 'pull' and 'push' against resistance.

6. Wrist – ask the patient to hold hand up straight and push away/towards.

7. Ask the patient to squeeze your two fingers in his hand.

8. Ask the patient to spread fingers put and you try to push them together.

9. Coordination – 'finger-nose'. Check for dysdiadokinesia.

10. Reflexes

11. Sensation

12. Lower limbs – check tone by moving knee and ankle. Also, can lift leg off bed. If increased tone the whole patient will seem to move and not just leg.

13. Check power of legs by asking to lift straight leg up against resistance, push leg into bed while try to lift it up. Bend and straighten knee against resistance. Move foot towards and away (as if pressing pedal) against resistance. Big toe against resistance (S1).

14. Coordination – drive feet up and down legs when eyes closed.

15. Reflexes – as above. When doing reflexes, look at muscle belly and not just for movement.

16. Babinski reflex.

17. Sensation (as above). Place tuning fork on bony prominence.

18. Thank the patient and summarise findings.

EXAMINATION OF THE LOWER LIMBS IN A DIABETIC

1. "Hello Mr/Mrs............. I am Dr. ...., SHO in this department. Because of your diabetes we need to examine your legs to make sure you do not have any complications from the diabetes. Please will you undress to your underwear. Nurse is here to act a chaperone."

2. Ask patient to walk; assess **gait**.

3. Ask patient to lie on bed and inspect legs: ulcers, gangrene, callus on soles, muscle wasting, hair loss and signs of infection. Look especially on soles and ankles. Ask patient "do you get a sensation on your feet as if you are waling on marbles/cotton wool?"

4. **Feel** legs for pain, temperature.

5. "I would like to examine your **pulses** now." Palpate pulses – femoral, popliteal, p. tibial and d. pedis.

6. 'Can I check your **sensation** now?' Check touch (cotton), sharp (disposable pin), temperature (hot/cold), vibration (tuning fork) and joint position.

7. Assess motor function – tone and power.

8. Check **reflexes**

9. Ask patient how often he/she visits the chiropodist.

10. Tell examiner that you would also like to check b.p., fundoscopy and HBA1c levels. Also, check injection sites if diabetic and look at their glucose monitoring book.

11. Summarise findings and thank patient.

THYROID EXAMINATION

1. Approach patient from RIGHT hand side; patient sitting in chair.

2. Introduce and ask for permission "I am Dr ___, How are you today? Is it OK if I examine you? You will have to take your shirt/blouse off. Is that all right? Do you require a chaperone?"

3. Hands – any fine tremor? hot/cold? (NB: Anxious-sweaty/cold, thyrotoxic-sweaty/hot.)

   Nails –olinichia?

4. Pulse – tachycardia?

5. Eyes – look from front for bulging, symmetry, infection, chemosis. Bottom eyelid should be bottom of iris and top eyelid at top of pupil. Any hairloss?

   Thryotoxic = lid retraction = eyes wide open

   Proptosis = Graves = bulging eyes

   Check eye movement – stand away from patient and hold patient's head with one hand. Hold the other hand about 1 foot (arms length) away. Show one finger to patient and ask: "Can you see my finger?"

"How many fingers can you see?"

   Then lean forwards and backwards – right to left – fingers held vertically. Ask patient to follow finger. Ask any pain?

   Also, move finger up and down and ask same.

Lid lag – hold finger horizontally and move slowly from top to bottom. Eyes and eyelid should move together. If the patient has lid lag, then eyelid lags behind eyeball.

Look from back when patient has head extended, i.e. looking at ceiling. Look for any bulging of eyes.

6. Neck –

Look at patient from front. Check for any masses in neck. If there is a swelling and you want to check if this is thyroid, ask patient to take a sip of water and swallow while you are looking at patient's neck. (NB: A thyroglossal cyst would also move on swallowing but it will also move when protrude tongue out, thyroid gland will not move with tongue.)

If masses, check:

Site

Size (about .... × .... cm)

Consistency (soft, firm or stony hard)

Surface texture (smooth-regular or irregular)

Mobility (freely mobile or fixed to surrounding tissues)

Temperature

Palpate thyroid gland from patient's back. Find thyroid gland with fingers of both hands. (NB: Thyroid gland is below the thyroid cartilage.) Once found, just feel the surface and edges with both hands. Then press down one side to steady gland while palpating the other. Swap over. (Just below the thyroid cartilage is thyroid isthmus.) So find the thyroid cartilage and move down and you will come to the thyroid isthmus.

Auscultate, listen at sides, don't press too hard. Use bell or diaphragm. You may hear the carotid and thyroid. To check whether bruit is from carotid and not thyroid then listen at a slightly higher position, i.e. angle of jaw. Here any bruit will be from carotid.

8. Ask patient to cough/say something – recurrent laryngeal nerve palsy

7. Reflexes – in hyperthyroidism get hyper-reflexia. In hypothyroid get normal reflexes but there is slower relaxation. Best place to check is ankle.

8. Check for pretibial myxoedema.

9. Thank the patient.

** You may be asked if you think patient is hyper/eu/hypothyroid. suggest what you think depending on findings. But always say I would confirm by blood tests tfts.

OPTHALMOSCOPY

Introduce yourself and explain to patient that due to the nature of their problem, you need to look at the back of his/her eye. Explain that you will use an instrument called an 'ophthalmoscope' and that you shall have to shine a bright light into patient's eye. Due to the nature of the test you shall have to get quiet close and also put your hand on their forehead. Mention you can use tropicamide 0.5% (work in 20 mins, last 8 hrs). Small risk of bringing on angle closure glaucoma.

1. For examination of the right eye sit or stand on patient's right.
2. Select '0' on the dial. If you know the patient's glasses prescription, then you can adjust the dial. If wearing contact lenses, there is no need to adjust dial – start at '0'.
3. Dim the room and ask patient to concentrate at an object in the distance, e.g. picture on the wall.
4. Hold the ophthalmoscope in your right hand (when testing right eye). Place your right index finger on the dials.
5. Hold the ophthalmoscope around 6 inches in front and slightly to the right of the patient and direct the light beam into the pupil. A 'red reflex' should appear as you look.
6. Rest the left hand on the patient's forehead. This gives you an idea of how far or near you are to the patient in the dark. While patient

holds fixation on the object, keep the 'red reflex' in view and slowly move towards patient. The optic disc should come into view when you are around 1–2 inches away from patient. If it is not then you need to adjust the lens so play with the dials. NB: The far-sighted patient needs higher 'plus' (black numbers) while the near-sighted needs more 'minus' (red) strength of lens.

Look at the lens and focus on colour, elevation and vessels. To find the macula move the light approximately two disc diameters in the temporal direction (outwards).

To look at macula, ask patient to look straight into light.

7. To examine the left eye, repeat the procedure as above but hold ophthalmoscope in left hand, stand on patient's left and use your left eye.

8. Summarise findings to examiner.

Slides possible in the examination

Abnormal pigmentation: Commonest is that with senile macular degeneration. Here get pigmentation around macula and everything else looks normal.

Optic atrophy: Disc looks pale. It is normally associated with decreased vision.

Papilloedema: Disc is swollen. Get congested veins and small haemorrhages. Get in raised intracranial pressure. It is normally bilateral here.

Retinal artery occlusion: Retina is pale (ischaemic) and macula looks 'cherry red'.

Retinal vein occlusion: 'Stormy sunset'. Cotton wool spots and flame haemorrhages.

Diabetic retinopathy: Dot/blot haemorrhages and microaneurysms. Signs of retinal ischaemia – cotton wool spots (look like bits of cotton wool), new vessels and venous dilatation. Affects vision. Treat new vessel growth with photocoagulation. Remember annual eye checks in diabetics.

Hypertensive retinopathy: Arterio-venous nipping, i.e. crossover of arteries over veins. Flame haemorrhages, hard exudates (yellow caused by lipid leakage). Hypertension rarely affects vision.

EAR EXAMINATION – OTOSCOPY

1. Greet and introduce yourself to patient. Say "Due to the nature of your problem we need to examine your ears with an 'otoscope'. It is uncomfortable but not painful. If it hurts, please let me know. You will have to keep still. "If examining a child, then ask the mother to keep the child on her lap with one side facing her. Ask her to hold the head still while you examine ears.

2. Check equipment is working and get appropriate sized speculum.

3. Look at the pinna and surrounding skin. Look for any deformities. Make sure you look behind the ear for any swelling or bruising.

4. Now slowly insert the otoscope and examine the external ear canal. The best view in a child is achieved by retracting the pinna backwards and in an adult retracting the pinna upwards and backwards. NB: Hold the otoscope like a pen, i.e. between thumb and index finger with the ulnar border of hand gently resting on patient's face.

5. After examining the external canal, look at the tympanic membrane. Normally the tympanic membrane is semitranslucent and grey. NB: If there is a lot of wax then I would ask patient to use something like olive oil for a week and then have ears syringed. I would

like to see him after he has had this done to make sure that the drum is fine.

6. Thank the patient and explain findings to examiner.

Common Abnormalities

External ear: **Otitis externa**. Hurts when you pull pinna. Pus or debris in external ear. Redness in outer ear. More commonly you will see wax.

Serous otitis media: There's increased vascularity of the drum and it loses its colour. Loss of cone of light. May see fluid level behind drum.

Acute otitis media with or without effusion:

Here the drum is congested with blood vessels. The ear drum is bulging outwards. May see fluid level behind the drum. Also, look for perforations.

Perforation of drum: Quite obvious. They need antibiotics and referral to ENT as an outpatient.

Grommets: Like a plastic tube. Used in treatment of mid ear problems. Patients can swim but have to protect ears. Usually, fall out themselves.

CHEST PAIN AND MI ADVICE

Here the scenario may be

- Manage a patient who has been admitted with central crushing chest pain into your A&E department.
- Look at this ECG and make diagnosis and treatment options (MI, AF, VT).
- Advise this gentleman who has had a MI regarding lifestyle changes.
- Explain the following anti-anginal medications.
- This gentleman has a strong family history of IHD. What advise will you give him?

1. Chest pain patient in A&E

- Introduce and greet
- Chest pain – start, last, intensity, type, radiation, ass. symptoms
- NB: If lasts >20 mins ass. with nausea/ sweating and not made better by GTN then this is probably not just angina
- PMH/DH

Examine: Does he look ill?
           BP/Pulse/Sats
           ECG

Signs of heart failure, arrthymias

Treatment: PAIN RELIEF – i.v. diamorphine 2.5 mg – 5 mg with maxalon 10 mg
             Aspirin

Oxygen

?Thrombolyse – criteria

- New LBBB
- ST elevation of 1 mm in two consecutive limb leads
- ST elevation of 2 mm on two consecutive chest leads
- ST depression V1-V2 (i.e. post-MI)
- CCU

Investigations

Troponin at 12 hrs (generally >0.04 is significant)

CXR

Routine blood – FBC, UEs, cholesterol, glucose

NB: The ECG is the most important investigation. Should be done first at the same time as giving analgesia, taking blood, etc. Ask nurse to do ECG while you are doing above. This is because the quicker you diagnose a MI and treat the less myocardial damage.

You must learn the criteria for thrombolysis and the contraindications. Have you heard of bolus thrombolysis? may be given by trained paramedics.

2. Advise this gentleman who has had a MI regarding lifestyle changes

"Hello, Sir, is it OK if I talk to you about your illness and some lifestyle changes that will benefit your health?"

Start by saying "When you came in 2 days ago with chest pain, we diagnosed a heart attack. You also received treatment for this. A heart attack happens when one of the blood vessels supplying your heart gets blocked. For this reason you get the pain."

"There are a few things that you can do to prevent this happening. I will explain these to you:

Diet : Eat more fruits and vegetables and less fat, e.g. chips, meat. Eat chicken and fish. Reduce weight.

Exercise : You need regular exercise to train your heart and improve fitness. You need to gradually build up exercise, i.e. start with walking first, then jogging, then swimming. I will refer you to our exercise programme.

Smoking : You should stop smoking. We can give you advise phone number for this.

Alcohol : Restrict to 1–2 glasses a day of wine.

Sex : You can have it but as sex increases work-load on the heart, it may cause chest pain (angina). Taking a GTN tablet before hand may help, stop if pain starts.

Driving : Can start after 4 weeks but at first do short runs with friends.

Work : Depending on type of job can go back in 4-12 weeks.

Air travel : Avoid for 6 weeks."

3. Explain the following anti-anginals to patient

"The ones you need to know are:
- Aspirin
- GTN spray/tablets

- Beta-blockers
- Anti-cholesterol (statins)

Aspirin (show bottle) Take once a day with food. Can cause stomach irritation so, if does, let us know. We can change to different one or add something to protect your stomach. It works by preventing blockage of blood vessels.

GTN spray/tablet You spray or put tablet underneath your tongue. You only need to use it if you get pain in chest called *angina*. Always take it while sitting. Can cause headache, dizziness. You can get patches that contain the same drug as well. You need to change them everyday and also need to keep take them off for a few hours each day.

Beta-Blockers These tablets slow the heart down and reduce the work-load on your heart. They have to be taken regularly everyday. Do not stop. Main side-effects are it can drop your blood pressure and cause dizziness. May cause bad dreams or wheeze.

Statins As well as reducing the amount of fat and cholesterol you eat we will give you tablets to reduce it. Most of these have to be taken at night. Very few side-effects – main one it can affect your muscles of your body but this is rare. We will do blood tests to make sure this has not happened and also that your liver tests are normal."

4. Family history of IHD

The patient will come to you concerned asking what he can do to reduce his chances of IHD.

- Go through all the lifestyle changes
- Go through all risk factors
- Ask you will measure cholesterol, glucose
- Take aspirin
- See every year for above

Explain to him that IHD does tend to run in families.

Explain to patient that he is not showing any signs of IHD. However, it is important to treat any risk factors he may have. Also, he must adjust his life-style to reduce his risk.

ASTHMA GETTING WORSE

Scenario is young girl who has had asthma since a child but she is needing more inhalers now.

Take history

- How long have symptoms been getting worse.
- Anything making worse, e.g. pets, moving home, weather, cold.
- How regularly using inhalers and Check technique.
- What treatment is she on.
- Any cough, SOB, chest pain.
- Any previous admissions for asthma, any ICU admissions specifically.
- Normal PFR, what is it now.
- Smoking.
- Needing to take time off work/school.
- Does it affect sleep. Does she wake up in night SOB?

You need to find the precipitating factor. Could be pneumonia or moving house, or exam stress?

Treat cause

Does she need admission?

Treatment for acute exacerbations is generally:

- Oxygen
- Nebulised salbutamol 5 mg and ipratropium bromide 500 mcg (at least 4 × daily)

- Prednisolone 30–40 mg (NB: Hydrocortisone 200 mg i.v. can also be given but oral prednisolone is as effective)
- Antibiotics, if signs of infection
- If not better with above, move to i.v. salbutamol (5 mg in 500 ml N. saline – 30–90 ml/hr) or i.v. aminophylines.
- Notify ICU if getting tired

Investigations

- FBC, UEs, allergy tests, i.e. IgE to cats, dust, etc.
- CXR – exclude pneumothorax
- PFR
- Blood gases

NB: COPD management is similar but do not use high flow oxygen.

PANIC ATTACKS AND PALPITATIONS

You will most likely be given a young woman who gets above symptoms. Your job is to rule out any organic causes, e.g. arrhythmias, valvular heart disease, thyroid problems, etc. Then you should reassure the patient and provide advise.

Questions to ask

- "Describe the symptoms you are having.
- If palpitations, can you tap out rhythm – regular/irregular?
- Any other symptoms – SOB, chest pain?
- What brings your symptoms on?
- What relieves symptoms?
- Any weight loss, sweating, bowel change – symptoms of hyperthyroidism?
- Any symptoms of diabetes?
- Tremor?
- How much coffee, tea you drink?
- Cigarettes or any other drugs?
- Any signs of depression – appetite, sleep, mood?
- Suicidal thoughts?
- Past history including mental illness."

Examine thoroughly and do ECG and blood tests (FBC, UEs, TFT, LFTs and glucose).

Once ruled out, all organic causes explain that her symptoms are probably related to her getting worked up in certain situations. What she can do about it?

Explain to patient

"Mrs ____, listening to your symptoms it seems to me that most of your symptoms are caused because of your nerves. You are getting worked up in certain situations and the way your body reacts to this is by getting palpitations. This is an exaggeration of a normal body reaction. There are a few things that may help:

- Lifestyle changes – stop smoking, reduce alcohol, coffee, etc.
- Relaxation therapy – sports, yoga, music, etc.
- Try to avoid these situations that cause you to get worked up.
- Cognitive and behavioural therapy.
- Medications, e.g. propanalol? antidepressants, I would not suggest benzodiazepines as they can become addictive."

TIA or STROKE PATIENT

You may be given a patient who has had a stroke/ TIA, and asked to take a history and reach diagnosis. Then counsel patient for it.

NB: If you get a young patient with sensory loss or visual symptoms, make sure you exclude multiple sclerosis.

Things important in history are

- How long symptoms lasted?
- Past/family history.
- Any risk factors - diabetes, smoker, IHD, hypertension, cholesterol?

Explain to patient the diagnosis, i.e. he/she had a TIA/CVA which occurs if a blood vessel in the brain gets blocked.

Say "we cannot do anything to reverse it but we can help you to improve your weakness (explain physiotherapy, occupational therapists, specialist stroke wards).

Also, we need to prevent this happening again. This is done by treating all the risk factors that you may have:

- Stop smoking
- Exercise regularly
- More fruit and vegetables/less fat. Fish once a week.
- Loose weight

- Aspirin 75 mg regularly – warn them of indigestion, if history of ulcer don't give or can give antacid with it
- Cholesterol lowering drugs, e.g. statin
- Treat hypertension
- ACE inhibitors shown to provide some prophylactic benefit.

HEADACHE

Types of scenario:

1. Young girl on the OCP who is getting migraines
2. Cluster headache in mid-aged man
3. SOL headache with nausea
4. Tension headache and depression

1. Young girl on OCP getting migraines

Take history

What type of headache and where – throbbing, tight band around scalp?

How often – everyday, related to menses, work?

How long last?

Any warning?

Any associated symptoms – flashing lights, visual disturbance, weakness?

Any nausea?

Headache worse in any certain position, worse by coughing/sneezing?

Is it worse in mornings?

What have you taken for it?

Any trauma?

Any fever?

Any family history of migraine?

The patient will give symptoms of classical migraine, i.e. visual symptoms followed by unilateral headache, lasting a few hours. Occurs every month since on OCP.

Explain to patient that you think she has migraines. This is a common cause of headache and it is not associated with anything serious

Explain to the patient that the OCP is probably making the migraine worse. It is a known side-effect.

For this reason it may be worth trying a different type of contraceptive, e.g. progesterone only pill, IUCD, condoms, etc. Note that a normal migraine is not a contraindication to OCP, only focal/hemiplegic migraine is, can discuss treatment of migraine, e.g. analgesia with antiemetics (migraleve); or prophylactic drugs, e.g. propanolol, etc.

2. Young girl comes to you thinking she has a tumour

Questions

What type of headache and where – throbbing, tight band around scalp?

How often – everyday, related to menses, work?

How long last?

Any warning?

Any associated symptoms like flashing lights, visual disturbance, weakness?

Any nausea?

Headache worse in any certain position, or while coughing/sneezing?

Is it worse in mornings?

What have you taken for it?

Any visual symptoms?

Any galactorrhoea?

Any trauma?

Any fever?

Any family history of migraine?

Any weightloss?

Any FH of cancer?

Any fitting/drowsiness?

What are you worried about?

All the answers will be negative so reassure:

"Miss ____, after listening to your symptoms, I would reassure you that I do not think you have a brain tumour or anything sinister like that. It is more likely you are having tension headaches and because you are worrying about them they are getting worse.

With headaches caused by brain tumours it is generally worse in the mornings or on bending or sneezing. They also cause nausea. Brain tumours are rare but tension headaches more common.

I think we should treat you with simple pain-killers first. However, if you get any of the symptoms such as nausea, visual problems or drowsiness, you need to come to see a doctor immediately.

If your headaches do not improve, I will refer you to a specialist.

Do you understand? Do you agree? Any questions?"

3. SOL with nausea, etc.

The patient is 22 yrs and has been out with friends yesterday. He has been drinking and may have been in a fight. He has come to you requesting some analgesia. He has been sick twice this morning.

Take a history

He explains he has had sickness twice but this can happen after binging anyway. Feels more tired than normal. He lives on his own. Says the headache is worse after sneezing.

Say to him:

"Mr _____, your headache seems to be different than your normal migraine, do you agree?

You are also getting sickness and tiredness with it plus as you think you have been in a fight yesterday, I think we should send you to the hospital for some tests.

I think you may have something called a extradural haematoma, which is a blood clot around the brain. If it is this, you will need urgent treatment. It can be diagnosed easily by doing a scan. Also, treatment would be possible by surgery.

Do you understand? Any questions?"

Get an ambulance for him.

4. Tension headache and depression

This patient is a middle-aged woman with three children. Her partner has left her.

History

She explains headache is like a tight-band around head. Worse at end of day. No other symptoms except tiredness.

Talk to her and ask her specifically for:

Signs of depression:
- Sleeping
- Appetite
- Weightloss/gain
- Palpitations, etc.
- Suicidal thoughts
- Past psychiatric. History

How is she with children:
- Any help?
- How old are they?
- Any thoughts about injuring them?
- Any finance problems?

Explain to the patient you think her symptoms are related to her life. Explain that it must be difficult to bring up three young children on her own. The headache she describes is related to tension and stress. Also, she is showing some symptoms of depression. You would like to put her on anti-depressants. Explain it takes some time for them to start working and to persevere with them. Will need to be on them for at least a few months. Ask het to try some lifestyle changes like going out, seeing people. Get relatives/friends to help with kids.

You will like to see her again in 3-4 weeks to see how is she getting on.

"Understand? Any questions?"

5. Subarachnoid

Mid-aged businessman with severe headache. No past history.

Take a history after introducing yourself.

Patient says worse headache ever, like being hit in back of head. Feels sick as well.

Explain to patient that you think he may have something called a subarachnoid haemorrhage. This is bleeding from one of the blood vessels in the brain. It is serious and requires immediate attention. Say you shall organise him to be transferred to hospital by ambulance. There he will have a scan of his head, called CT and if diagnosed he will need operation.

Give nimodipine to prevent spasm of vessels.

Enquire if the patient has any questions?

EPILEPSY

With this you may get a number of situations, some possible ones are:

- Epileptic attack comes in fits – treat
- Somebody has been diagnosed with epilepsy – explain the implications
- Explain drugs for epilepsy
- Febrile convulsion (see paediatric Bit)
- Epilepsy getting worse

1. Epileptic fit management

As always ABC first – oxygen high flow, naso-pharyngeal airway unless trauma and basal skull fracture queried.

IV access and benzodiazepam – see flow chart 1 (on page 60).

Check that there is no history of trauma or fever (meningitis).

Check blood, esp. for glucose, UEs, calcium.

If stops, put in recovery position.

If status quo and not stopping, call anaesthetist - ICU.

2. Explain implications of epilepsy

Patient has been diagnosed with epilepsy already so you need to talk about what this means to him and treatment. What lifestyle changes he must make?

Chart 1

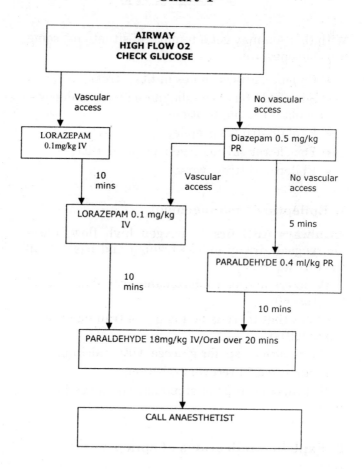

NB: If a person only has one fit then he is NOT diagnosed as epileptic but will not be able to drive for 1 year and also advise regarding working on heights, swimming alone, etc. If first fit happens after the age of twenty, you would suggest a CT scan to exclude SOL. Prior to this then EEG would be useful.

Explain to patient that she has been diagnosed with epilepsy. This means that she is prone to have seizures/fits. Explain that most of the time we do not have a reason why it happens but have ruled out serious things like tumour.

Drugs: Explain that she has been started on a tablet called _____. (Learn about Phenytoin, Carbamazepine and Valproate — Side-effects). "You have to take the tablet regularly and cannot stop. The tablets have to be taken a few times a day. These tablets can make the oral contraceptive pill and other tablets less efficient so she may need a higher dose of it or something different for contraception. Some tablets we have to monitor levels to make sure there is enough in blood. We may reduce the tablets after two years if she is fit-free."

Driving : Explain because of epilepsy, she cannot drive until she is fit free for one full year. If she was only getting fits during sleep, then this pattern has to have been for three years. For public service vehicles, e.g. HGV, buses rules are even stricter. All this is because of safety for herself and others in case she has fits while driving. Also, her insurance is void.

Wear **identity bracelet** stating she is epileptic.

Sports Never swim on her own or do dangerous sports on her own.

Work Should not work at heights or with heavy machinery.

Holidays Take enough medicine. NB: Carbamezepine can make hypersensitive to sunlight so extra cream and long sleeves. Also, avoid going out at noon. Be aware disco lights may start a fit so don't stay there for too long. Alcohol can affect the concentration of the drug in your body and can provoke a fit.

Pregnancy Most of the antiepileptics can affect the baby while it is developing. If you are thinking of having a baby then speak to your specialist. You will need to take folic acid. Also, do not just stop your medication as your epilepsy can get out of control otherwise.

LET PEOPLE KNOW YOU HAVE EPILEPSY

3. Epilepsy getting worse

Scenario is that a patient comes to you stating her fits are more often and lasting longer.

In history ask:

- Are you on medication and which ones
- Compliance
- Any stress
- Fever/illness
- What is bringing fits on
- Alcohol? Any other drugs
- Any injury – head
- Sleep deprivation?

WEIGHTLOSS

Usually you will be given a scenario in which young girl presents with weightloss

You have to split this into organic problems (e.g. hyperthyroidism, chronic diseases, diabetes) and psychological illness (e.g. anorexia, depression)

Ask

- When noticed weightloss?
- How much over what period?
- Any palpitations – other hyperthyroid symptoms?
- Any night sweats?
- Any change in bowel habit?
- How is your appetite?
- How are your periods?
- Any medication?
- Any stress at work/school/home?
- How is your sleep?
- How is mood – feeling low?
- How is concentration?
- Do you enjoy things that you did in the past?
- Do you think life is not worth living?
- Suicidal thoughts? – "Have you thought about harming yourself?"
- Are you exercising too much?
- Do you make yourself vomit?
- Do you think that you are thin/overweight?

Once you have excluded all serious organic causes explain that you think her weight loss is related to depression and not eating properly. Go through treatment options, e.g. antidepressants. Length of time she needs to be on and that it takes a while for it to start working.

If thinking along lines of anorexia then explain that this is a disease and that it can be serious. Say that as her weight is so low it will affect normal body functioning such as her periods. Also, it can cause serious abnormalities in blood tests (do UEs). You will refer to dietician and psychiatrist and they will monitor her weight.

NB: If young patient brought in by relative then more likely to be things like anorexia. If come themselves then more likely organic cause.

ANALGESIA

The type of scenario possible is some guy with terminal cancer needing analgesia. Also, you could be given a lady who has become constipate from morphine use.

1. Talk to the wife of Mr Jones who has cancer regarding analgesia

What you have to go through:

- Introduce and say sorry to hear your husband has been diagnosed with cancer. Explain one of his problems may be pain and we can do something about this to keep him comfortable.
- Start with paracetamol first – can take two tablets four times a day. Very few side-effects unless taken in o.d.
- Then can give anti-inflammatories if no contraindications, e.g. asthma or ulcers. Explain there's ones like ibuprofen – take two four times a day. Very good for bone pain. Main side effect is that it can upset stomach and cause indigestion/ulcers. If this happens tell us and we will stop. NB: COX II inhibitors may be better.
- Then onto opioids – start with weak opioids such as dextroproproxyphene and then move to stronger, e.g. codeine and morphine. Explain side effects, i.e. Constipation, nausea (can give antiemetic), drowsiness and risk in o.d. Explain can take when needed but best to take slow

release preparations regularly and then small doses on prn basis.

Make sure she understands everything. Answer any questions and say you will go through it again if needed.

2. Mrs Billington has been admitted to the ward with abdominal cramps. AXR confirms constipation.

Make sure you have ruled out any other cause for the pain before you blame it on constipation.

Treatment options:
- First you have to treat the acute problem and then do something to prevent it happening again.

    PR suppositories (glycerine). Try up to two and if fail move to things like phosphate enema. Again try up to two if fail then a bit stuck. Options include things like microlax and picolax. They come in sachets and never use a full one on elderly. It can cause dehydration, etc. Be careful if use and also ask senior before using.

    Prevention – things like SENNA and LACTULOSE on a regular basis. There are also things like bisacodyl, etc. Also, what caused the constipation in the first place, e.g. diet – improve it – more fibre, etc. If on morphine – does she need to be on it? Can we change it?

DIABETIC KETOACIDOSIS MANAGEMENT

Scenario a patient is admitted with severe dehydration and drowsiness. He is diabetic.

Severity assessed by:

- Conscious level
- Degree of dehydration
- Degree of acidosis

Mainstay of treatment is treating dehydration aggressively and giving insulin.

On admission:

- I.V. access and take bloods for FBC, UEs, glucose, venous bicarbonate
- Blood Gases
- Urine for ketones
- CXR
- Blood cultures
- MSU
- ECG and cardiac enzymes if over 40 yrs

Start fluids:
- 1 litre N. saline stat
- then, 1 litre over 3 hours
- Add potassium

PLASMA K	DOSE TO ADD
<3.5	40mmol
<5	20mmol
>5	None

NB: If patient is elderly or has heart disease then infuse fluid at half above rate

GIVE INSULIN according to **sliding scale**:

BMs	INSULIN/hr
0-5.9	1/2U
6-9.9	1U
10-13.9	2U
14-17.9	3U
18-20	4U
>20	6U + CALL DOC.

To make dilute 50 units of soluble insulin (eg. actrapid) in 50 mls of N. saline. Use N. saline as infusion fluid for dehydration treatment. However, if BMs <15 then switch to 5% dextrose.

Can switch to subcutaneous insulin once patient is ketone free and eating/drinking.

Bicarbonate is very rarely needed to treat the acidosis. The rehydration normally also treats acidosis. If thinking of giving then speak to senior first.

NB: Subcutaneous heparin may need to be used especially in HONK cases.

NB: Find the cause for the dka, e.g. infection, cardiac event, etc.

FEVER

Scenario could be a person with temperature for two weeks. Take history and give differential diagnosis.

Your aim is to pin-point the specific system that could be affected, e.g. resp., malignancy, abdo. Etc.

NB: Post-op. temp. could be wound infection, haematoma, DVT/PE, abscess, etc. Treatment is usually blindly started with augmentin or cef/met. combination.

Questions to ask

- How long had temp.
- Any night sweats
- Any rigors (causes of rigors Ascending cholangitis, pyelonephritis and malaria)
- Cough, phlegm
- UTI symptoms
- Weightloss
- Travel abroad
- Job, e.g. risk of legionnaires, etc.
- Any medication

Investigations

- FBC, UEs, LFT, ?cardiac enzymes
- Blood cultures
- MSU
- CXR
- Sputum

- Wound swab
- ?Malarial screen

Also, read the **PYREXIA OF UNKNOWN ORIGIN** section in Oxford Handbook of Medicine

JOINT PROBLEMS

May be given a range of scenarios:

- Young person with trauma and ankle injury
- Alcoholic with gout
- Rheumatoid arthritis
- Other connective tissue disorders
- ALWAYS CONSIDER SEPTIC ARTHRITIS IF ONE JOINT AFFECTED

Questions:

- Which joints
- For how long
- Are they getting better/worse
- Any other symptoms, e.g. swallowing problems, skin problems
- Any bowel problems
- Any trauma
- PMH/FH
- Any drugs
- Alcohol hx
- Is pain worse at any time
- Any STIFFNESS
- Any penis discharge, sexual activity?

If considering things like rheumatoid arthritis or gout do the appropriate blood tests:

- FBC
- UEs/LFT

- CRP/ESR
- Rheumatoid factor
- Urate
- Tests for SLE, etc.
- XRAYs

For trauma patients, e.g. sprains:

DVT/PE

May get given scenario where you take history and diagnose either. Note to diagnose you need to do:

DVT: venogram or Doppler

P.E.:   VQ scan or spiral CT (if CXR is abnormal then better than VQ)

NB: it may take a few days to get above investigations so you would say that you shall start treatment prophylactically anyway. If they are haemodynamically unstable after PE then consider ICU and thrombolysis.

Go through risk factors:
- Immobility
- Previous thrombosis/family history
- Trauma
- Smoking
- Oral contraceptive pill
- Protein C + S deficiency, Factor V Leiden, anti-phospholipid, etc.
- i.v. drug user

Another possible scenario is advising someone who is concerned about thrombosis and wants advise regarding travel.

Say that the main cause of DVT from flying is because of immobility. That is if you are on a long haul flight and do not keep moving then your blood circulation is slower esp. blood returning from your legs and this increases thrombosis risk. If you have had multiple thrombosis in past you should be on prophylactic warfarin. If no history of thrombosis, then advise:

- Stay active
- Drink plenty of water
- Specialised stockings may help
- ?Stat dose of aspirin
- Ff any symptoms, e.g. calf pain or chest pain/ SOB see doc.

POST-MORTEMS AND DEATH CERTIFICATES

Death Certificates

To fill in death certificate, one must be:

- A qualified medical practitioner and must be the doctor looking after the patient.
- He/she must have seen the patient in the last 2 weeks or after death (if someone else been looking after during the past 2 weeks).
- He/she must know the cause of death.

Writing Death Certificate

1a Immediate cause of death, e.g. myocardial infarction.

1b Main disease causing the death, e.g. coronary thrombosis.

1c Underlying cause, e.g. ischaemic heart disease.

NB: You do not need to fill all 3 sections.

2 Other diseases contributing to death, e.g. diabetes.

Post Mortems

When is it a legal requirement:

- When the dead has not been seen by a doctor in the last disease.

- Cause of death is not known.
- Not seen in the last 14 days by any doctor.
- Suspicious circumstances, e.g. violence/neglect.
- Industrial causes.
- Poisoning (NB: alcohol is not seen as a poison).
- Death during surgery or before recovery from anaesthetic.
- Accidents.
- Death in police custody.

Scenario: You may get is talk to son of Mr Bob who died suddenly two days after a hip replacement. He did have IHD.

Introduce yourself and say "I am sorry about your father. I would like to discuss a rather delicate matter with you. As you are aware your father was doing quite well after the operation, however, unfortunately yesterday he developed chest pain and passed away. We did everything possible but could not resuscitate him.

As everything has happened suddenly we do not know the cause of death. Therefore, we need to do something called a post mortem."

"This is a legal requirement and not something we can decide. It is like a surgical procedure and done by specialist doctors. They will look inside your father's body and look specifically at the organs such as heart. Usually the body leaves some clues of what caused the death.

We will not remove any organs and disturb the body as little as possible. Everything will be put back as normal but he will have a scar along his body.

If we can find out what has caused his death then we may get clues of how we can prevent a similar thing happening in the future with relatives. The whole process takes a few hours.

You can start making preparation for the funeral."

"Any questions?"

- If the son is against post-mortem, you have to tell him that it is a legal requirement and not something you can decide. It may benefit his relatives if we can prevent the same happening to someone else.
- What is he worried about? e.g. removing organs, etc.

COMMUNICATION

MEDICAL/SURGICAL HISTORY TAKING

Be polite

"Hello, my name is Dr _____. Is it OK if we talk about your health?"

First get to know patient's full name and age.

Occupation at present.

PC: The problem in patient's own words, e.g. back pain, etc.

HPC: Go in detail into the problem.

Specifically how long had it, ever had it before?

Any other symptoms?

Pain – type, site, severity, radiation, ass. symptoms, ever had before, constant.

Cough – sputum, SOB, wheeze, worse with activity

PMH: Any other medical problems in past, e.g. diabetes, heart problems.

PSH: Any operations in past.

DH: List of drugs taking. Any Allergies.

SH: Smoker?

Job?

Alcohol

FH: Any illnesses in family?

ROS: Quick run through all systems, e.g.

CVS	:	palpitations, chest pain, faints
Resp.	:	SOB, asthma
GI	:	weight loss/gain, change in bowel habit, pr blood, jaundice
G.U.	:	periods, UTI
CNS	:	headaches, CVA/TIA, epilepsy

In the end ask

"Have I missed anything or is there anything else you would like to add?"

"Is there anything specific you want to say/ ask?"

PHONING FOR ADVICE

Some important points

- Know the patient information which you will need.
- Are you asking for advise or do you want your senior to come to see the patient? Be specific.
- Apologise for disturbing.
- Only give relevant info. – PC, relative PMH, examination findings, obs, what you have done.
- Let them ask questions.
- Make sure you understand info. given.
- Are you happy with info. given or do you want your senior to see patient themselves?
- Say "Thank You."

Examples

1. You are on the surgical ward. A young girl has been admitted with signs of obstruction. She has had previous bowel operations. You think she needs to be seen by a senior.

You: "Hi it's Sanjay speaking, sorry for disturbing you."

Reg.: "No worries, what the problem?"

You: "I have just seen a 20 yr old girl who has been admitted via A&E with vomiting and abdominal pain. She gives a two-day history of severe abdominal Pain, gradually increasing severity. She is requiring morphine at present. She's been vomiting profusely. Examination shows that she looks dehydrated, b.p. is 90/50 and pulse 125. Abdomen is hard with some voluntary guarding. Rest of examination is normal. The AXR confirms small bowel obstruction. This girl has had a bowel operation for Crohn's and I think she has obstruction secondary to adhesions."

Reg: "I agree. Have you put n.g. tube."

You: "Sorry, yes I have and she also has a drip going. I have sent blood samples for FBC, UEs, LFTs and amylase also, Plus G+S."

Reg: "Great. That should do."

You: "Thank you, but I think it would be good if you see her when you have time."

Reg: "I'll be right there."

2. **Another example could be a nurse ringing for advise, e.g. a post-op. patient who spikes a temp. and b.p. has dropped.**

Important things

- When they ring you up, say you will be there in 2–5 minutes. Tell them where you are at present.

- When on ward, find the nurse that bleeped you. Ask her if anything has changed and ask her to accompany you while you are seeing the patient.

- Once you have seen the patient, say what you think is going on, e.g. "I think this gentleman has an infection somewhere."

- Tell her what your plans are now, e.g. "I will take blood for FBC/UEs/blood cultures/G+S. Also, we will start a drip Hartmans."

- "I will let the registrar know."

- "Please keep a close eye on urine output."

- "I will come back to review in ½ hr but bleep me if needed."

- "Do you agree with the management?"

CONSENT

The following information has been taken from the GMC guidelines.

Introduction

1. **Respect patients' autonomy, their right to decide whether or not to undergo any medical intervention,** even where a refusal may result in harm.

2. **Find out what the patients want to know and ought to know:**

- **details of the diagnosis, and prognosis**, and the likely prognosis, if the condition is left untreated;
- uncertainties about the diagnosis, including options for further investigation prior to treatment;
- **options for treatment or management** of the condition, including the option not to treat;
- the purpose of a proposed investigation or treatment; and
- **benefits and the probabilities of success**.

3. You should raise with patients the possibility of additional problems.

4. **You should not withhold information necessary for decision-making unless you judge that disclosure of some relevant information would cause the patient serious harm**.

5. No-one may make decisions on behalf of a competent adult.

Ensuring voluntary decision-making

6. It is for the patient, not the doctor, to determine what is in the patient's own best interests. Nonetheless, you may wish to recommend a treatment or a course of action to patients, but you must not put pressure on patients to accept your advise. In discussions with patients, you should:

- give a balanced view of the options;
- explain the need for informed consent.

You must declare any potential conflicts of interest, for example where you or your organisation benefit financially from use of a particular drug or treatment, or treatment at a particular institution.

Children

7. You must **assess a child's capacity to decide** whether to consent to or refuse proposed investigation or treatment before you provide it. In general, a competent child will be able to understand the nature, purpose and possible consequences of the proposed investigation or treatment, as well as the consequences of non-treatment. Your assessment must take account of the relevant laws or legal precedents in this area. You should bear in mind the following:

- At **age 16,** a young person can be treated as an adult and can be presumed to have capacity to decide.
- **Under age 16, children may have capacity to decide, depending on their ability to understand what is involved:**

- Where a competent child refuses treatment, a person with parental responsibility or the court may authorise investigation or treatment which is in the child's best interests. The position is different in Scotland, where those with parental responsibility cannot authorise procedures a competent child has refused. Legal advise may be helpful on how to deal with such cases.

IN SUMMARY

- Know about the procedure you are consenting patient for. If you are unsure, ask first.
- Explain everything in lay terms so that the patient understands.
- Provide all relevant info. so that the patient can make informed choice.
- Use pictures/models wherever possible.
- Explain why the patient is having procedure in first place.
- What are the alternative options available.
- Go through all common complications. Also, explain the potential serious complications.
- Nobody can consent for (another) mentally competent adult.
- For children, those under 16 yrs can consent if mentally competent.
- Under 16 yrs cannot refuse treatment. If they do, then involve their parents.
- Let patient ask questions and make sure they have understood everything.
- If in doubt, ask seniors.

EXAMPLE

1. You are the HO and need to consent a patient for hernia operation. It will be done with local infiltration but tell patient of different options, e.g. spinal or general.

You: "Hello Mr Jones, my name is Dr _____ and I will be looking after you while you are in hospital. Is it OK if I talk to you about your operation?"

Mr Jones: "Hello, yes please do."

You: "Do you know what operation you are having and why?"

Mr Jones: "I've got this hernia and it needs putting back in place. How it's done I have no idea."

You: "No problem Sir, I will explain you everything. Also, you need to sign this consent form at the end."

Mr Jones: "No problem"

You: "You have this lump down below which is a part of your bowel. There is some weakness in the muscles there and so this bit of bowel is in the wrong place. The operation you are having will repair this weakness.

First it is important that you are aware that this operation will be done while you are **awake**. However, we shall give you pain-killing injections so that you do not feel anything. If you do not like this idea then we can ask the anaesthetist to give you a general anaesthetic so that you sleep during the procedure or you can have an injection in your spine to make everything numb, below waist.

What will happen is that you shall be changed into theatre clothes and taken to theatre. In the theatre a doctor called an anaesthetist (specialist in this) will inject a local anaesthetic around your groin. This will numb the area so that you do not feel them operating. They will make sure that the area is numb before they start but if you feel anything you just say. You should not feel pain but will feel some touch or pulling.

Once the area is numb, the surgeon will make a cut along your groin (point to part of body). It will be around 5 cm in length. Then he shall move the tissue and muscle that is underneath the skin out of the way.

Once he sees the hernia, he will push it back into its place and put a mesh over it. The mesh will make the muscle walls in your groin stronger and prevent the hernia coming back.

The surgeon will then put the muscles and skin back in place. You will have some stitches or staples. These will be removed in 5 days.

Do you understand everything until now?"

Mr Jones: "Yes."

You: "That's good. Like any other operations there are some potential risks with this operation. The main side-effects are infection, bleeding, failure to repair the hernia completely. Also, there is a very small risk that your bowel or some other organ can be damaged. This is extremely rare but as it is serious, we have to mention."

Mr Jones: "Yes, I understand."

You: "Good, will you sign this consent form which explains what you are having and why. And that I have explained everything to you. Also, it is important that you have the option of not having this operation. This, however, has the risk that this hernia may get bigger and may twist and cause severe pain and emergency surgery."

Mr Jones: "No, I'll have the operation."

Put consent form with notes, give patient a copy. Check heart/lungs and make sure he is fit for operation. Ensure that he had the routine blood tests done?

BREAKING BAD NEWS

THERE IS NO RIGHT OR WRONG WAY

Who Does It?

Should be done by the most appropriate person. Not necessarily a doctor; could the nurse looking after the patient.

STEPS

Before

- Refresh yourself with **WHO** the patient is and **WHAT/HOW** he/she died.
- Which relatives and how many are going to be there.
- Have you or anyone met them before and what have they been told.
- Find appropriate room, e.g. relatives room. Must be a **quiet place** where you cannot be disturbed but found if necessary.
- Tell people where you going and for how long.
- Get colleague to hold bleep if possible.

Meeting

- **Introduce** yourself and get to know how relatives are related to the patient.
- Say how you are involved with patient care.
- Ask them what they already know.
- Say "Mr/Mrs — has passed away/died".

- Give brief description of what happened.
- If talking about terminal cancer, tell also what you can do, e.g. pain-relief, McMillan nurses, hospice care.
- Do they **understand?**
- Any **questions?**
- Ask you will be willing to meet again if they would like.
- Tell them what happens now, e.g. Death certificates coroner's involvement, etc.
- **Document** your conversation.

NB: **Pauses** are extremely important to allow people to take things in and also think and understand.

EXAMPLES

1. Patient passed away after unsuccessful CPR

You are going to speak to Mr Blogg's daughter and wife. They are waiting in the relative's room for you. They know that Mr Bloggs has had a cardiac arrest but not the outcome. You have been looking after Mr Bloggs for the past few days. He was a 80 yr man admitted with pneumonia and has arrested. CPR was done for 20 minutes but no success.

Before you see them you read his notes and get Sister James to accompany you. You have told other staff where you will be and have given your bleep to your HO.

You: "Hello Mrs Bloggs, my name is Dr ____, and I have been looking after your husband over the past few days and this is Sister James. Is this your daughter?"

Mrs Bloggs: "Yes. What's happened doctor?"

You: "As you are aware, Mr Bloggs was admitted with a severe chest infection. At his age a simple infection can be difficult to treat and sometimes too excessive for the body to cope with. Unfortunately, at around 4 pm, Mr Bloggs' heart stopped beating. We tried to resuscitate him but unfortunately failed. Mr Bloggs has passed away."

Pause (let them say the next thing)

Mrs Bloggs: "Did he suffer?"

You: "We do not think so. Prior to this happening he was comfortable."

Mrs Bloggs: "He never complained anything, he was very nice. What happens now?"

You: "You can go and see him if you like. I will sort out his death certificate and sister here will explain to you the procedure. I am happy to see you again if you like. If there are any questions, you can ask to speak to me or any of the staff."

Mrs Bloggs: "Thank you doctor."

2. Telling someone they have cancer

Mr Jones is a 50-yr old plumber. He has smoked all his life and recently admitted with haemoptysis. His CXR showed a suspicious lesion which has been confirmed by CT/biopsy to be lung cancer. He does not know anything yet. He is on his bed.

You read through his notes and scans. Take a nurse with you and see him in a side-room, if possible.

You: "Hello Mr Jones, my name is Dr _____, and this is staff-nurse Ann. I would like to talk to you about your investigations. Is that OK? Would you like anyone to be with you at present, e.g. a relative?"

Mr Jones: "Yes, please doc. I've been worrying all along. Is it bad?"

You: "Mr Jones, would you please tell me if you have been told anything yet?"

Mr Jones: "They've seen this shadow on the x-ray but not said anything."

You: "Mr Jones, you came to us with coughing blood. For this reason you initially had a CXR. This showed a sinister looking shadowing. We needed to find out what this could be, so we organised other tests. Unfortunately, the scan and biopsy have confirmed that it is lung cancer."

Pause

You: "Do you understand Sir?"

Mr Jones: "Yes, I thought it could be cancer. What does this mean now?"

You: "Because of where it is, it may be possible to remove it by surgery. I will refer you to a specialist who after seeing you and the scans will decide. If this is not possible, we could send you for radiotherapy. However, at all times we would want to treat any symptoms you may have, e.g. if you have pain we can give you pain killers."

Mr Jones: "Thank You"

You: "Have you understood what we have spoken about? Would you like to ask any questions?"

Mr Jones: "No doc. You have explained it well. Thank You."

You: "I am available to speak to you again if needed. Once I know more about your referral, I will let you know. Do you want me to tell your relatives if they ask?"

Mr Jones: "No please don't. They will just worry. I will tell them."

DOCUMENT IN NOTES WHAT YOU HAVE TOLD HIM

3. Mr Bob is dying of terminal gastric cancer. He wants you to speak to his wife who is his main carer.

Again you take with you a nurse after the reading notes. Again in relatives room.

You: "Hello, Mrs Bob, my name is Dr _____, and I have been looking after your husband. This is sister June. I would like to have a talk about your husband Mr Bob. Is that OK? Would you like anybody with you?"

Mrs Bob: "Yes, doc. Please do."

You: "What have you been told about your husband up till now?"

Mrs Bob: "I've been told he has cancer in the stomach and this is what he will die from."

You: "Yes, Mrs Bob. Your husband does have cancer of the stomach and unfortunately it has reached a stage where we can no longer treat. However, there are many things we can do to make things comfortable. Such as pain killers, feeding him through a drip and helping him feel more comfortable. There are also some specialist nurses called McMillan nurses who can give you advise."

Mrs Bob: "Yes, that would be nice. How will these nurses help?"

You: "They can advise you and provide support. They will also be involved with pain relief and helping with sickness. This is because some strong pain-killers cause sickness. They can also help to get some financial benefits to help you look after your husband."

Mrs Bob: "How long do you think he will live?"

You: "It is very difficult to predict this. People vary from each other."

Mrs Bob: "Can I take him to a hospice?"

You: "This may be possible. However, we will look into this for you."

Mrs Bob: "Thank You"

You: "Is there anything else you want to ask? Have you understood everything?"

Mrs Bob: "Yes, thank you."

You: "I am happy to see you again to keep you updated."

Document above

In the above scenario it is important to mention what you can do, e.g. pain-killers, emotional support, etc. Also, **McMillans nurses'** role is vital.

SURGERY

ABDOMINAL PAIN

Possible scenarios

- **Right upper quadrant pain**
- **Right iliac fossa pain (appendix)**
- **Epigastric pain**
- **Acute abdomen**

Questions

- All the pain questions, i.e. where, type, radiation, ass. symptoms, etc.
- Weight change
- Change in bowel habit
- Nausea, temp. (appendix)
- Urine/stool colour (gall stones)
- Any chest symptoms (right upper quad., pain could be due to pneumonia)
- Any chance of diabetes (DKA can cause abdominal pain)
- Any foods make it worse (e.g. fats and gall stone pain)
- Sickle disease
- ?MI

Acute Abdomen

If asked to see then similar to above but here history is less important. Things to do:

- Check obs. – b.p./pulse/temp.
- Insert 2 X cannula and take blood samples for FBC, LFTs, amylase, blood cultures, cross match 4 units, clotting screen.
- Catheterise – strict input/output balance.
- i.v. Hartmans
- AXR + erect CXR
- Inform Registrar and operation theatre
- Cef. + met.
- ECG, if elderly

PR BLEEDING/CHANGE IN BOWEL HABIT

Possible scenarios

- Young chap with pr bleeding noticed on wiping. Advice regarding piles and lifestyle.
- Mid-aged with blood mixed with stools – possible cancer.
- Loose stools + mucus in young girl. ? Crohns
- Weightloss–problem with absorption, e.g. coeliacs.

Questions

- How long been bleeding
- Is blood mixed with stools or fresh
- What colour are stools
- Any mucus
- Any weightloss
- Is stool difficult to flush away
- Any pus
- Any night sweats/temp.
- Any PMH/FH
- Any sensation of still wanting to, after you been already (tenesmus)
- Any lumps/prolapse
- What are your worries
- Travel abroad
- Any vomiting
- Anyone else in family affected
- Any rash/eye problems

HAEMATURIA

Possible scenarios

- Young person with flank pain and symptoms of ureteric colic
- Elderly with frank haematuria – rule out malignancy
- Secondary to rifampicin or excess rhubarb
- Unlikely to get things like Goodpasture's, etc.

Questions

- How long had it
- Any pain
- Weightloss/night sweats
- Stones in past
- PMH/FH
- Any drugs
- History of polycystic disease
- Any UTI symptoms
- Travel abroad

Investigations

- FBC, UEs, LFTs
- KUB Xray
- MSU
- Bone profile
- Urate

- G+S
- IVU
- Cystoscopy
- Counselling if find polycystic kidney disease

SCAPHOID

History

- Fall onto outstretched hand may lead to fractured scaphoid. But it can also lead to fracture at wrist, radial head and humeral neck.
- May get a mixture of fractures.
- Even suspect scaphoid fracture get x-ray; ask for scaphoid view.
- Treat as if fracture, i.e. scaphoid plaster for two weeks.

Signs

- Tenderness in anatomical snuff box.
- Pain on ulnar deviation of hand.
- Compression of thumb leads to pain., i.e. push thumb into it's socket leads to pain.
- Tenderness over thenar eminence (site of scaphoid tubercle).

Management

- If suspect scaphoid plaster (NB: will cover half of thumb and below elbow) and review in two weeks with repeat x-ray.

NEEDLESTICK INJURY

In Hospital

- Risk is low.
- Treat all blood contact as infected.
- Needlestick wound should be encouraged to bleed straight after exposure. Do not suck wound.
- Wash with soap and water.
- Report incident to senior doctor/nurse. Contact occupational health and fill in the adverse incident form.
- Take 10 ml blood from patient to check for infectivity. Take 10 ml blood from victim for storage. May need to test for infection later.
- If fully immunized for hepatitis B, there is no need for prophylaxis. If not immunized and if the patient is known to have hepatitis B, then you require hepatitis B immunoglobulin within 72 hrs as precaution.
- Check tetanus status.

In Community

- Take 5 ml blood for storage.
- Start course of accelerated (0, 1, 2 months) Hep B vaccine if not immune.
- Check tetanus status.
- Reassure that risk of HIV is very low but if the person is concerned, counselling and HIV testing at 3 months can be offered.

ABDOMINAL EXAMINATION

1. Approach patient from right hand side.

2. Introduce and ask for permission "I am Dr ___, how are you today? Is it OK if I examine you? You will have to take your shirt/blouse and trousers off. Is that all right?" (In the exam you will just ask the patient to move trousers lower so that you can see hernial orifices, there is no need to take off trousers completely.) Ask for a chaperone.

3. Examine hands – **nails** (kolynichia, clubbing, temp., sweating, etc.)

4. Check eyes – jaundice, anaemia, arcus.

5. Check mouth – tongue, teeth.

6. Check neck for lymph nodes.

7. Look at abdomen – scars, symmetry, masses, pulsations. Get to level of abdomen and watch.

8. Ask patient "Are you sore anywhere?" (Always start away from that point.)

9. **Gentle palpation**: Start from left iliac fossa, then to left subcostal and flank. Moving to right subcostal and then iliac fossa. While palpating ask the patient to breathe in and out. Look at patient's face for any signs of pain. Any guarding, rebound tenderness or rigidity.

10. **Deep palpation,** i.e. in same areas but firmer.

11. **Liver:** Palpate on right side at level just above umbilicus. First gently and then more

firmly. Ask patient to take deep breaths in/out. When breath in the liver moves down. Move up from level of umbilicus.

Percuss liver again from level of umbilicus and moving upwards until above liver, i.e. into lung.

12. **Spleen** – Start at below umbilicus. Put right hand under the right subcostal region and palpate with left hand. Move towards spleen while palpating. Ask patient to breathe in/out.

13. Left **Kidney** – Put left hand into loin (back of kidney area). Use right hand to feel, i.e. balloting kidneys. (NB: Breathing does not move kidney.)

For right kidney same but put left hand into right loin.

14. **Bladder** – Percuss area of bladder.

15. **Hernial orifices** and ask patient to cough while checking.

16. Palpate femoral pulses and aorta for aneurysm.

17. Percuss for **ascites**. Also, shifting dullness or fluid thrill.

18. Auscultate for bowel sounds (wait for at least 3 minutes before decide 'no bowel sounds'). Auscultate around renal arteries for bruit.

19. Ask patient to stand and check for hernia.

20. Say to examiner "I would like to do a pr and genetalia examination" (in males).

21. Thank patient.

TESTICULAR EXAMINATION

1. Get consent from patient, i.e. tell him that "due to the nature of your complaint I have to do an examination that will involve examining your groin region. Is that OK? It will not be painful but may feel uncomfortable. I am going to ask staff nurse here to chaperone, is that OK? I have to do most of the examination while you are standing."

2. Expose area, i.e. take trousers down and look for any lumps, bumps, colour changes, infection, etc. Feel hernial orifices and check for impulse.

3. 'Now I am just going to make sure there are no abnormalities on your penis.' Get hold of the penis and look at the top surface, then bottom surface. Look for ulcers, cancer, infections, etc.

4. Retract foreskin and look underneath foreskin. If there is any discharge, send it for culture.

5. Raise scrotum and look at rectal area for fissures, tags, prolapsed haemorrhoids, ulcers, etc.

6. Look at undersurface of scrotum.

7. Feel both testicles with two fingers to see that they are the same size. Check that they are both there. Ask if there is any pain.

8. Feel testes with thumb and finger for any lumps, etc. Slide any lump between finger and thumb. Feel for lumps on the top and

bottom surface and at the top and below. Lumps you may find are:

- Spermatocele
- Testicular tumour
- Epididermal cyst
- Hydrocele

9. Transilluminate testes and any lumps. Lumps that illuminate are hydroceles.

10. Ask patient to cough and look for an impulse, i.e. lump gets bigger.

11. Do hinge test to check if you can get above the lump. Do this by putting finger at the top of the scrotum and lifting scrotum up. If it is a pure testicular lump, then you can do the hinge test easily. If the lump is not purely in the scrotum, e.g. inguinal hernia, then hinge test is difficult. Do hinge test on both sides of the scrotum.

12. Feel regional lymph nodes and pulses.

13. Say "I would like to do a pr examination now" to check prostate, etc.

RECTAL EXAMINATION

1. Get consent from patient, i.e. tell him/her that "Due to the nature of your complaint I have to do an examination that will involve examining your back passage. This will involve inserting my finger into your back passage. Is that OK? It will not be painful but may feel uncomfortable. I am going to ask staff nurse here to chaperone. Is that OK?"

2. Get patient into correct position. Ask him/her to lie on his/her left hand side, come as close to the edge of the bed as possible. Bend knees up to the chest, hips at 90° and knees bent to 110°. Ask "Are you comfortable? Try to relax and take deep breaths in and out."

3. Look at rectal area for any fissures, tags, haemorrhoids, ulcers, cancers and infections. Look also for blood and mucus.

4. Wear gloves and get some lubricant gel.

5. From the side, insert your index finger gently feeling for the anal sphincter. Ask patient to squeeze or 'bear down' so that you can check rectal tone. If there's increased tone it is probably due to anxiety. If there's both increased tone and pain then it's probably an anal fissure.

6. Move up pressing backwards.

7. Once right up feel for any masses posteriorly. If there is a mass work out whether it is

outside or inside the lumen. Soft, hard, smooth, fixed? Can you feel the sacrum?

8. Turn finger to patient's right side and feel for caecal or appendix masses.

9. Turn finger anticlockwise to left side of patient and feel sigmoid colon. Faeces will be indentable.

10. Turn finger forwards to feel prostate in males and cervix (feels like tip of nose). Make sure prostate is not tender. Then feel for the lobes and then the groove. Feel for any lumps. If feel a lump say "I can feel a lump in the right lobe.' Describe the site, size (eg pea size), consistency (soft/ hard), surface (regular/ rough).

11. Gently withdraw finger out and look on finger for any mucus, blood, etc. Send sample off for an occult blood test.

12. Thank the patient and ask him/her to get dressed. You will come and explain the findings to him once dressed.

ASSESMENT OF THE ARTERIAL SYSTEM

Possible scenario is "examine a diabetic foot" or "assess the circulation in this patient". In the first one it is important you check sensation, etc. In the second case you have to assess venous function as well. Get permission and ensure privacy. Get chaperone.

1. Look at colour of skin, any hair on legs, gangrene, etc.

2. Find **Buerger's** angle. This is the angle to which the legs must be raised before they would turn white. Normally even at 90° legs still stay pink. Once the legs have gone white or fatigued, ask the patient to sit at the edge of the couch with legs hanging (**Buerger's test**). Watch the feet for a few minutes. If the test is positive, i.e. vascular insufficiency, then they will become cyanotic-red and if normal they will stay red.

3. Check **capillary refill** time. Put slight pressure on nail bed for 2 secs. See how quickly it returns to pink again.

4. Is there any venous guttering, i.e. collapsed veins.

5. Look at the pressure areas for any ulcers/ sores. The main ones are heel, malleoli, head of 5th metatarsals, toe.

6. Palpate skin – is it warm?
7. Check pulses – femoral, posterior tibial, popliteal and dorsalis pedis.
8. **Auscultate** for bruit over aorta, iliacs and femoral pulses.
9. Measure blood pressure in both arms to exclude subclavian vessel narrowing – get difference in b.p. You also get difference in b.p. with aortic dissection and to differentiate between the two you can do a CXR or Doppler of subclavian artery.
10. Thank patient and explain findings.

EXAMINATION OF THE VENOUS SYSTEM

1. Explain to the patient "Because of the nature of your problem I need to examine your legs. Will you please undress to your underwear. Nurse here will act as a chaperone."

2. Ask patient to stand up and look for any veins. Any oedema, eczema, pigmentation or ulceration.

3. Feel at the sapheno-femoral (2–3 cm below and 2–3 cm lateral to pubic tubercle) and sapheno-popliteal junction for a cough impulse. A strong cough impulse means incompetence at these valves.

4. Tell the patient that you would like to do a special test (**Trendelburg's Test**) so that you can find where the abnormal veins are. "I will lift your leg up and empty your veins in your leg I will then apply pressure on your thigh where I think there might be a problem. I will ask you to stand up at this point and see if you get your varicose veins again."

   Lie the patient flat and then elevate one leg until all the blood from the superficial veins has drained. Once it has all drained, place pressure over the sapheno-femoral junction and ask the patient to stand up while you are doing this. See if the veins fill up while you are applying pressure. Release pressure and see what happens. If the sapheno-femoral junction is incompetent then the veins will only fill when pressure is removed. Tell examiner that you can do a similar test using tourniquet.

5. **Percuss** over vein, and if a vein is incompetent and distended you will get a positive percussion impulse. Put on finger at the base of the vein (lowest part that you can see) and tap at the upper part of the vein. A positive test is when you can feel an impulse at your finger which is at the bottom of the vein.

6. **Auscultate** over vein cluster to listen for an arterio-venous fistula.

7. Thank patient and explain findings.

CERVICAL SPINE EXAMINATION

The examination of the spine may be asked. Usually it is the lumbar spine. Easiest way to remember the system is thinking in your head what movements can I do with this joint, e.g. neck – you can look up (extension), down (flexion), sideways (rotation) and touch your shoulder with your ears (lateral flexion). You won't be expected to know exact percentages of movement but more whether you think they are restricted or painful. Look slick and you'll get away with most things! Always, **l**ook, **f**eel, **p**assive **m**ovement and then **a**ctive **m**ovement.

1. Introduce yourself. "Hello, my name is Dr _____. I am the SHO in A&E. Is it OK if I examine your neck? Please, just loosen the top few buttons of your shirt so that I can get a good look. Does it hurt anywhere?"

2. Look for obvious deformities, e.g. torticollis (wry neck) due to muscle spasm, loss of lordosis (rheumatoid arthritis), increased lordosis (ankylosing spondylosis).

3. Get permission to feel the neck: "I'm just going to feel your neck now. Is that OK?" Feel for any bony tenderness and then feel along muscles for tenderness. The main muscles are the trapezius and the paraspinal.

4. Now "I am going to ask you do move your neck, I will tell you exactly in which direction." Look for symmetry of movement.

- "Look to the right and then to the left" – rotation-80°
- "Tilt your head to the right and then left, try and touch your shoulder with your ears" – lateral flexion – 45°
- "Look up to the ceiling" – extension – 60°.
- "Look down at the floor" – flexion – 75°.

5. Perform passive movement. See if range of movement is greater than active movement.

6. Check upper limb reflexes and ask the patient if he/she has any sensory symptoms, e.g. pins and needles.

7. Thank the patient and summarise findings.

THORACIC SPINE

1. Introduce and ask the patient for permission to examine his/her back. "Please can you undress to your waist." Get chaperone. Examine patient standing.

2. Inspect the spine from the front, back and sides. Look for any deformity like kyphosis or scoliosis.

3. Tell patient that you will be touching patient's back. Feel the bones for any tenderness. If there is no tenderness then percuss the bones with your fist or tender hammer.

4. Ask patient to sit on a couch as this will stabilise the pelvis. Look for any deformities. If scoliosis is present, ask patient to lean forwards. See what happens to the deformity. If scoliosis was due to abnormal posture or muscle spasm, it will disappear.

5. Ask patient to "please turn to the right and then left."

6. Measure chest expansion; normal is 5 cm or more.

LUMBAR SPINE

"Hello, Mr/Ms _____, my name is Dr _____. I am the SHO. Because of the nature of your problem I need to examine your lower back. Please, will you strip to your underwear? (get a chaperone). Can you stand up for me please?"

1. Look from behind and side. Look for any scoliosis and check if the lordosis is normal.

2. Palpate over the bones and ask for any pain? Also, check over paraspinal muscles.

3. Ask the patient to bend sideways.

4. Ask the patient to bend backwards and then forwards. Keep knees straight.

   Schober's test (checks for flexion problems) – make a mark at dimple of Venus. Make another mark 5 cm below this and one 10 cm above the dimple of Venus. Place tape measure on lower mark and ask patient to bend forwards. Note how much the upper mark has moved. Normally the upper mark should increase by 5 cm. Reduced in alkylosing spondylosis.

5. Ask patient to walk and assess gait. If there is disc prolapse then patient will lean to the opposite side.

6. Now you need to check for nerve compression. The ones you check are sciatic (L4–S1) and femoral (L2–L4).

Sciatic

Straight leg raise: Patient should be lying supine. First you need to check that hip flexion is normal. Do this by lifting leg up while knee is bent. Then extend knee and raise the leg up straight. Note the angle at which it hurts. Ask patient is this the problem you were telling me about? At the angle when pain is felt dorsiflex the ankle (Bragaards test) – this will increase the pain if there is nerve root compression.

Bowstring test: Do straight leg raise as above. When the patient complains of pain, flex the knee and pain should disappear. Now start extending the knee again until pain returns (Lasegue's test). Another test is the Bowstring test. Here apply pressure with thumb in different parts of the popliteal fossa. First nearest to the examiner, then in middle and then over hamstring tendon. A positive test is when the second bit is more painful.

Sitting test: Only a patient who does not have sciatic nerve irritation can sit up from lying position without help.

Flip test: Get patient to sit at the edge of a table/couch so that legs are hanging off bed. Knees are at 90°. Tell patient that you are checking ankle reflex. Extend the knee gently. A person with true sciatic problem will flip backwards due to pain.

7. Check ankle reflex and strength of dorsi-flesion of big toe. Check sensation.

8. Say to examiner that you would like to do pr for rectal tone and check for sacral anaesthesia.

9. **Femoral**: Ask patient to lie prone and then gently flex the knee until get pain. If this does not cause pain, then extend hip while knee is still flexed.

10. Examine sacroiliac joints by applying firm pressure with the heel of the hand over the sacrum.

EXAMINATION OF THE HAND

1. "Hello, my name is Dr _____. I am the SHO. Because of the nature of your problem I need to examine your hands. Please will you roll your sleeves up of both arms."

2. Inspect hands for any wasting, deformities (e.g. swan neck), lumps, scars. Look for any subcutaneous nodules, e.g. Herbedon's. Is the skin warm, any colour change (Raynauds)? Any nail changes, i.e. clubbing, splinter haemorrhages.

3. Palpate the joints and check for tenderness or swelling. Feel for any lumps on the tendons as patient is flexing and extending fingers.

4. Check movement:
   - Pinch with two fingers (best thumb to little finger)
   - Put hands in prayer position and then lower hands while keeping palms together, checks wrist dorsiflexion.
   - Put back of hands together and raise arms, checks wrist flexion.
   - Ask patient to flex DIP joint while holding finger in extension at PIP, checks the FDP (flexor digitorum profundus).
   - Ask patient to flex PIP against resistance while others in extension, checks FDS (flexor digitorum sublimes).
   - To check median nerve, ask patient to abduct vertically upwards the thumb against resistance.

- Ulnar nerve – ask patient to hold card between the fingers and thumb. If there is weakness, the thumb cannot be held straight and flexes.

5. Asses patient's neurologic and vascular status.

READ UP ON SOME COMMON DEFORMITIES, e.g. Boutonnieres, mallet finger, etc.

? Carpal tunnel syndrome

There are two tests. You may get scenario of a patient who has it clinically.

It occurs due to compression of median nerve in the carpel tunnel. Get paresthesia and numbness in the thumb, index and half mid finger. In **Phalen's** test flex wrist for two minutes and you get the pain patient has been complaining. **Tinels** – you percuss over carpel tunnel. This should lead to pain if positive test

SHOULDER EXAMINATION

1. "Hello Sir. My name is Dr ____. Is it OK if I examine your shoulder? Please take your shirt off please. Where is the pain. Is it worse on movement?

2. Inspect – look at shoulder from back and look for asymmetry and muscle wasting.

3. Palpate along muscle and joints (acromo-clavicular and sternoclavicular) for any tenderness.

4. Ask patient to place hands at the base of neck. Ask patient to reach from the bottom from behind and try to touch shoulder blades.

5. Ask patient to move arms forwards as if marching, checks flexion.

6. Ask patient to abduct arm. If the patient cannot start abduction, then he has rotator cuff rupture – he will be able to abduct if you do the initial abduction for the patient. While abducting, ask if there is any pain (due to impingement). If there is pain, check for painful arc syndrome. If the patient gets pain between 40°–120° this is in subacromial bursitis, supraspinatus tendenitis and supraspinatus tendon tear.

7. Thank patient.

HIP EXAMINATION

1. Introduce yourself and explain to patient that you would like to examine the hip. Explain that he/she will have to strip to the underwear. Get chaperone and ensure privacy.

2. Ask patient to walk – observe gait. Look for any tilt.

3. Do Trendleburg test to asses any abductor weakness. Get in arthritis, polio and congenital problem. Ask patient to stand on one leg and then the other with hands in front of them. You stand in front of the patient in case he/she falls. Tell patient "I will hold you if you lose your balance." If there is a problem, the pelvis tilts and the patient will lean over to the side of the lesion.

4. Get patient to lie on bed. Look for any weakness, muscle wasting, scars, lumps. Palpate for any tenderness over hip and pelvis (do splinting of pelvis).

5. Measure leg length – cross over legs and measure from anterior superior iliac spine to medial malleolus.

6. Movement – check flexion, i.e. move leg up. Normal = 120°. Check for any flexion deformity by doing Thomas's test. Put one hand on patient's back (lumbar region) and flex hip as much as you can until your arm is being squashed by the lumbar spine. If there is flexion abnormality then the opposite leg will flex off the bed.

7. To check for abduction/adduction, fix the opposite side of the pelvis and move hip in (adduct-normal 25°) or out (abduct-normal 45°).

8. Bend knee to 90° and rotate hip at pelvis to check internal (30°) and external rotation (45°).

9. Thank the patient.

KNEE EXAMINATION

1. Introduce yourself and explain to the patient that you would like to examine the knees. Explain that he/she will have to strip to the underwear. Get chaperone and ensure privacy.

2. While the patient is standing, look for any genu valgum/varum. Examine back of knee for Baker's cyst.

3. Get patient to lie supine on couch.

4. Inspect – weakness, wasting, effusions, scars, deformity, erythema. Measure muscle girth at 10 cm above patella – compare both sides.

5. Palpate along knee – any tenderness. Palpate along joint line too.

6. Movement – place one hand on knee and ask the patient to flex knee. Feel for any crepitus. Look for any flexion contractures.

7. Check for any fluid collection in the joint – squeeze above patella with palm of one hand, with fingers of opposite hand tap patella. If excess fluid feel tapping as patella hits femur.

    Massage test – massage any fluid from the medial side of knee into suprapatellar pouch (above patella), then massage the medial side and push fluid back into lateral part.

8. To check stability of knee, you have to check the anterior/posterior cruciates and collateral ligaments.

Collaterals: Extend knee and then flex ever so slightly. Hold ankle between your elbow and body. Gently abduct and adduct the femur and feel for laxity.

Cruciates: Flex knee to 90°; make sure hamstrings are relaxed first. For anterior cruciate hold onto tibia below the knee and pull forward. Check for laxity. For posterior cruciates you will see a sag while knee is flexed at 90°, also you can push backwards and feel for laxity.

(NB: Compare one side with the other.)

Another test is the **Lachman test** (see Macleods for more detail).

Pivot shift test is done as after some anterior cruciate injuries you get some complex rotatory instabilities. To do this, put one hand over the heel and the other just below knee. Int. rotate the foot and at the same time applying valgus strain at knee. Flex knee between 0 and 30° and feel for

9. Check if the patient has patella instability – patient is supine and knee extended. Push against the medial side of the patella and while maintaining this pressure, flex knee to 30°. Patients with an unstable patella would not let you do this.

To test for meniscal injury. These are bits of cartilage in joint. They can tear off and patient will complain of locking of joint in certain positions. For this do **McMurray test** – the knee and hip are flexed to 90°. Hold patient's heel with right hand and hold knee with left. Extend the knee slowly while feeling joint line with left hand. Do this with tibia in external rotation and then in internal rotation. If there is a problem then you feel a clunk.

10. Thank the patient and summarise findings.

* Ankle injuries – See booklet or course
* Blood forms, observation charts, etc. – See booklet or course

OBSTRETRICS AND GYNAECOLOGY

You will most likely get an obs. and gyn. scenario, which may be either as a communication and counselling station or as a practical OSCE. Possible scenarios are:

- **Perform a speculum examination and a smear**
- **Perform bimanual examination**
- **Breast examination**
- **Interpret and explain the smear result**
- **Counsel a woman who is 8 weeks pregnant and has pv bleeding**
- **HRT and contraceptive counselling**

HISTORY TAKING

PC: e.g. PV bleeding

HPC: through description of problem, including coital problems, e.g. dyspareunia. Ask "Is it affecting life?"

PMH:

Gyn. Hx: including last smear, last period, cycle length/regular, etc.

Obs. Hx: any children, mode of delivery (e.g. someone who has had 1 child and 1 miscarriage = G2 +1)

Contraception Hx:

SH: smoking/alcohol/job

DH: e.g. antiepileptics

ROS: as always

HRT ADVICE

A patient comes to you complaining of sweating and mood changes. You have done FSH/LH and oestradiol and have confirmed menopause. Talk to her:

"Hello, my name is Dr _____. Do you remember those blood tests that we did? They confirm that you are going through the menopause. Would it be all right if I talk to you about it?"

"The menopause is a time when your body slows down its production of female hormones. The main one is called oestrogen and it is produced by the ovaries. Oestrogen has actions all over the body. It maintains the skin texture and without it the skin becomes thin and dry. You get the same effect in the vagina where it causes dryness. Without this oestrogen, women start getting all the symptoms that you are having. These include sweating, mood changes, sleep problems, etc. A major problem with loss of the oestrogen is that your bones start becoming weaker. This is called 'osteoporosis'. With this you are more likely to get fractures.

One way of preventing all these symptoms is by having HRT. HRT contains oestrogen and also another hormone in women who have a womb. There are many ways in which you can have HRT such as tablets, patch, creams. Which one you wish to have is your choice. The tablets you have to take everyday, the patches you change twice a week and you have to apply creams daily.

HRT solves all the hot flushes and mood changes. It can take a few weeks for it to show full effect.

Some women are not suitable for HRT. These are those who have liver disease, cancer in the womb or breast. Also, if you are having abnormal bleeding down below then it is not wise to have HRT.

Like anything else, HRT also has a few side-effects. Most of them are minor and are things like sickness, weight-gain and some reactions to the patch. There is a small risk of breast cancer. However, in those who have been on HRT for five years the risk is minimal. However, once you get beyond using HRT for more than 10 yrs, the risk continues increasing. For this reason we advise women to stop HRT at 10 yrs.

It is important that you know that HRT is not a contraception and we advise women to continue with some contraception for 1 yr after the menopause."

CONTRACEPTION ADVICE

Possible scenario is to speak to a young girl who is asking for the pill, or discuss tubal ligation with this patient.

"Hello, Miss Blades, is it OK if I talk to you about the different contraceptive pills?"

"There are two types of pills, one which contains two hormones – oestrogen and progesterone. This is more popular. The second contains only one hormone – progesterone. This one is also known as the *mini-pill*."

The first one which has both hormones is very reliable. The failure rate is 1/100. It works by stopping the egg being released every month. It will also make your periods lighter and less painful.

The pill is taken daily for 21 days and stopped for the next seven days. You will get your period during these 7 days. It has to be started on the first day of your bleeding but if started after the fourth day then you have to use alternative contraception for 7 days.

If you forget it but remember in less than 12 hrs then that is OK. However, if it has been more than 12 hrs, then the pill may not be very reliable and you have to take extra precautions for the next 7 days. You also have to take extra precautions for 7 days if you have diarrhoea or if you are on antibiotics or some other drugs.

The main disadvantage with this pill is that it increases risk of thrombosis in the leg. Also, if you have any risk factors for heart disease you cannot take it. Also, if you have liver disease or some types of migraines you cannot have it. Smokers have to stop taking it at 35 yrs. It cannot be used when breast-feeding.

While on the pill you have to have your blood pressure checked every 6 weeks.

The second type of pill is the 'mini-pill'. This contains only one of the hormones (progesterone). This works by preventing sperm to enter the womb. It also makes it difficult for the womb to accept a fertilised eggs and in some cases even stops egg release (ovulation). It has to be taken at around the same time each day. This is also quite effective with a failure rate of 1/100. It is very useful for women who are older that smoke. It can also be use when breastfeeding.

The main side-effects are weight-gain and irregular bleeding.

If the tablet is taken three hours later than normal them it is not as effective and you need to use alternative means of contraception. Also, if you have diarrhoea then you have to use alternative contraception during diarrhoea and also for the following week."

?ECTOPICS

There is a lady who is 8/40 pregnant and has come with pv bleeding and pain. Take history and counsel.

"Hello, my name is Dr _____. Is it OK if I ask a few questions about what brought you to hospital?"

"When was LMP? Are they regular?

When did bleeding start?

Is blood dark or brown (ectopic) or is it heavy and fresh (miscarriage)?

Have you noticed any clots or anything unusual down below (e.g. products of conception)?

Where is the pain? Spread to shoulder?

Describe it (crampy with miscarriage).

What started first, the pain (ectopic) or the bleeding (miscarriage)?

Have you been using any contraception at present (e.g. coil)?

Do you have any children? Normal deliveries?

Have you ever had ectopic pregnancy? Have you ever had previous miscarriages?

Do you have any discharge down below? Does it cause any symptoms? Smell?

How are your bowels/waterworks?

Do you have any other illnesses? Do you take any medication?

Have you suffered any dizziness? Have you fainted?"

Examination: Obs., abdominal, pelvic, bimanual and speculum (swabs and remove any products if seen). Also, is cervix open?

Investigations: U/S pelvis, FBC, UEs, G+S, pregnancy test. Test, B-HCG.

Explain to the patient

"Mrs _____, you have come to us with some bleeding and pain. The most likely possibility is that you are having something called a 'threatened miscarriage". This means that there is a chance that this pregnancy may miscarry. This is not your fault and there is nothing you could have done to cause or prevent it. Around 20% of pregnancies miscarry early on. The thing that will help is resting.

There is a very slim chance that you may have something called an "ectopic pregnancy", have you ever heard of this?

In an ectopic pregnancy the fetus is lodged outside the womb. This is dangerous as it can rupture and bleed. We need to do a scan and this will give us a better answer. If it is an ectopic pregnancy you will need an operation. I would not worry about that at present. We shall talk about that once you have had your scan.

Do you understand? Any questions?"

THE LADY HAS HAD A SCAN, CONFIRMS ECTOPIC. COUNSEL HER REGARDING OPERATION

"Hello, Miss ____. I would like to have a chat with you about your scan. Is that OK?"

"When you came in, your main complaint was of pain and bleeding. We thought you may have something called an 'ectopic pregnancy'. The scan confirms that you do have this. Do you understand?"

"An ectopic pregnancy is one that has lodged itself inside the tubes instead of being in the womb. This is a dangerous situation because if we leave it as it is there is a chance it may burst and you can bleed heavily from this. Ectopic pregnancies never go to term and if we leave it then it is potentially life-threatening.

To treat it you require an operation. The operation can be done as keyhole surgery. You will have two cuts made on your tummy. One will be at the belly-button and the other below the bikini line. They will be both around 2–3 cm. We shall insert a camera into your tummy and remove the ectopic pregnancy. Because of the nature of the ectopic, we have to also remove a part of your fallopian tube. If we cannot do the operation safely by keyhole then we shall need to make a larger cut.

We shall try to save as much of the tube as we can. However, you can still become pregnant with only one tube.

Because you have had one ectopic pregnancy, you have a slightly higher chance of having another one again. What we would do is that when you become pregnant again we shall scan you early."

"Do you understand? Any questions?"
"You will be in hospital for 3 days."

LADY WANTS STERILIZATION – COUNSEL HER

"Hello, Mrs _____, my name is Dr _____. I believe you would like to have your tubes tied. Is that right?' May I ask you a few questions first?"

- "How old are you?
- How many children do you have? How were they born?
- How long have you been with your partner?
- Does he know of your decision? What does he think?
- Have you been on any other means of contraception? Which ones?
- Have you had any problems?
- Have you considered the depot injection/IUCD?
- Do you have any illnesses?
- Have you had any operations?"

Explain the operation

"The operation itself is quite simple and most people go home the same day. You will have a general anaesthetic. It can normally be done by keyhole if you have not had any operations before. You will have two cuts. One around the belly button and the other below the bikini line. They will be around 1 cm length. The surgeon will insert a camera and will find your tubes and clip them.

If it is not possible or safe to do the operation by keyhole then we will have to do something called a 'mini-laporotomy'. Here you would have a slightly longer cut around the bikini line.

Like any operation there are a few potential risks. The main ones are infection, bleeding. There is a very small risk of damage to other organs such as bowel. Also, having the tubes tied increases your risk of having an ectopic pregnancy if you became pregnant. This is the pregnancy lying outside the womb. There is a small failure rate as no contraception is 100%.

We would advise you to use some alternative means of contraception until your period after the operation.

It is very important that you treat this operation as Permanent, as the chances of reversal can be low. Also, you would not be able to have a reversal on the NHS. The advantages of tubal sterilization is that it does not interfere with your natural cycle and ovaries."

"We have to mention all the different options for contraception and the potential risks and you can make your own informed choice."

"Do you understand? Any questions?"

GENTLEMAN REQUESTING VASECTOMY – COUNSEL

"Hello Sir, my name is Dr ____. I believe you are considering having a vasectomy. Is it OK if I have a chat about it?"

- "How old are you?
- How many children do you have?
- How long have you been with your partner?
- What contraception have you tried?
- What does you partner think of your decision?
- Do you understand that this procedure should be viewed as permanent?"

"The operation is done under local anaesthetic. This means that you will have an injection down below which will numb the region. However, you will be awake during the procedure.

In the operation the tubes that carry the sperm are tied. The doctor will make a cut in the skin of the scrotum. He will look for the sperm tubes and cut a bit away. He will tie the remaining ends. The skin will usually be closed with 'butterfly stitches' (steristrips). You may require stitches but they will be dissolvable. They disappear in a week. The operation lasts only 15 minutes and you can go home. You should ask somebody to drive you home.

Like any operation there are potential risks. The main ones with vasectomy are infection, bruising and bleeding. If this happens, contact your GP or us. Wearing tight underwear for a day helps support the scrotum and reduce bleeding and pain.

Sex is possible as soon as you find it comfortable. However, you must use alternative means of contraception for 2–3 months. This is because you have sperm storages. We need two clear sperm tests so that you can safely rely on the vasectomy.

It is important you are aware that you will still continue producing male hormones and things like 'climax' will not be affected. The amount of secretions will be similar to before. You may have heard of a link between vasectomy and prostate or testicle cancer. However, this is not yet proven.

There is a very small failure rate of 1/1000–2000. You should treat this as PERMANENT as reversal can be dangerous and not 100% guaranteed. Also, a vasectomy does not protect against sexually transmitted diseases."

CERVICAL SMEARS

Possible scenarios are taking a smear and talking to someone who has an abnormal result.

Talk to this lady whose routine cervical smear shows severe dyskaryosis.

"Hello, my name is Dr _____. Do you remember the smear test you had earlier? I would like to talk to you about the results. Is that OK?"

"A smear is a test to make sure the cells at the tip of your womb, called the cervix, are normal. We can look for abnormalities and treat them before they become cancer. It is done every 3 years (NB: Some places, e.g. Manchester this is every 5 yrs) in women aged between 20 and 64.The smear result comes back as being either normal or abnormal. When it is abnormal it means that the cells have changed slightly but this is not cancer. Abnormal means that it is in between normal and cancer, but not cancer itself. That means that before you get cancer there are a number of stages and our aim is to catch the disease while it is in this stage so that we can prevent cancer. Do you understand?"

"Unfortunately, your result has come back in this region between normal and cancer. For this reason we need to have a closer look at your cervix. This is done by a process called 'colposcopy'. Have you heard of it?

For protocols – see booklet or course.

Colposcopy is done at the hospital. The doctor will insert a speculum down below, very similar to when you had a smear. He/she will then look at the area with the colposcope – it is like a magnifier. To get a better look he/she will apply some liquid to your cervix and will take a small sample called a biopsy. This might pinch a bit. This biopsy will go to the lab and we should get a result by 10 days.

After colposcopy you are advised to refrain from intercourse for 3 weeks. This is because there is usually a blood stained discharge. Also, use pads instead of tampons and shower instead of bathing.

Once we get the biopsy result, we can decide on what further treatment is required. This can be laser, freezing or cutting the abnormal area.

After the treatment, you shall be followed up with a second colposcopy at six months. This is to make sure everything has been cured.

Do you understand all of the above? Any questions?"

"As we have discovered these cells, we will be able to treat it. The chances of it spreading to cancer are minimal as long as you continue with follow up. You cannot spread the abnormal cells to anyone so continue enjoying sex."

STD

'Speak to this married lady who thinks she has a STD.'

"Hello, my name is Dr ____. How can I help you?"

"I think I have an infection down below."

"Is it OK if I ask you a few questions?"

- "How old are you?
- Have you noticed a discharge? Colour, smell, irritation?
- Any pain/bleeding with or after intercourse?
- What contraception do you use?
- Do you have a sexual partner? How many?
- Have you ever had a STD?
- Any children?"

Explain

"An STD is an infection that is spread by sexual intercourse if no protection such as condoms is taken. They are very common nowadays and many different organisms can cause them. Some of these you may have heard of such as *chlamydia* and *gonnorrhoea*. The symptoms you can get are discharge, bleeding, pain on intercourse and even no symptoms.

What will happen now is that we shall refer you to the GUM clinic. There they will take some swabs from down below. They will also check your urine and take blood. The whole procedure is fully confidential. We can give you the number of the clinic in this town but you can go to a clinic in any town.

We would advise you to tell your partner to go to the GUM clinic as well as he may be carrying the same organisms as well. He may not even have any symptoms. If you don't want to tell him yourself then the GUM clinic can send him an appointment inviting him to come. They won't tell him that you have been there."

"Do you understand? Any questions?"

"Here are some information leaflets."

TERMINATION OF PREGNANCY

Possible scenario is young girl who is 6 wks pregnant requesting a termination.

Termination of pregnancy can be done for the reasons mentioned in the sheet. Two doctors have to sign the 'Blue Form'. They have to both agree that the woman fits into one of the criteria as mentioned on that form. If a doctor, for ethical reasons, does not want to sign the form, then he/she does not have to. However, he must refer the patient to another doctor who will.

All termination of pregnancy cases are done in hospital – either medical or surgical.

"Hello, my name is Dr ___. How can I help?"

"I would like to have a termination."

"OK Can you tell me when your last period was? OK that makes you 6 weeks. Why do you think you want to have a termination?"

"I work and have to go to university. I think having a baby will make me very depressed. I will not be able to cope."

"Do you have any children?"

"No"

"Have you spoken to your partner about it, what does he think?"

"He agrees."

"Have you considered carrying on with this pregnancy and giving your child for adoption?"

"Yes, but I cannot do that."

"OK if you think a pregnancy will affect you psychologically, I am happy to refer you to the hospital for a termination. However, I need to discuss with you about contraception. What do you use at present? I can put you on the pill once you have your termination. Also, do you know that emergency contraception is available in case you have an accident in future? This can be taken up to 72 hrs of intercourse."

"Yes, I will go on the pill. Thank you."

"Any questions? I will refer you today and you should phone them in the morning to find out the date of your appointment."

"At the hospital they will examine you, including a speculum and do triple swabs (chlamydia, gonorrhoea and high vaginal). They will also organize a scan to confirm pregnancy and age. They will then discuss modes of termination. At six weeks gestation you could either have a medical or surgical termination. **I do not think you need to know the details of this.**"

PRE-ECLAMPSIA

This has been a new station. More of it is actually counseling the patients and telling them what it means and what will happen now.

'Talk to this 35/40 pregnant primip who has raised b.p at 150/110 and oedema.'

"Hello Miss ___, my name is Dr ____. Is it OK if I have a chat with you? Do you know that your blood pressure is slightly raised?"

"*Yes.*"

Questions:
- "Any headache?
- Any swelling?
- Any tummy pain?
- Any visual symptoms?
- Is you baby active?
- Any loss down below?"

"Because of the raised blood pressure and swelling around your ankles, I think you may have something called 'pre-eclampsia'. This is a disease that has many symptoms, some of these are high b.p. and swelling. It is serious and we need to admit you for observation and treatment."

"Do you understand?"

"The good thing is that your baby seems to be well according to the heart tracing (CTG). We need to admit you to hospital. There we shall check your b.p. regularly (every 4 hrs), check your urine, your baby and take some blood tests. These will give us a better idea of what is happening."

"Do you follow?"

"We may need to give you some tablets to regulate your b.p. These will not harm your baby. If your blood pressure does not get controlled on tablets then we may need to deliver your baby earlier. At 35 weeks the baby is very well developed and we do not anticipate any problems if delivered early. However, the children's doctors will want to keep you baby on the special baby unit."

"Do you understand?"

POST-NATAL DEPRESSION

A lady is brought to your surgery by her partner. She delivered 5 weeks ago and has been very low recently. Her partner is concerned she is not caring for the baby. Take a history and assess.

"Hello, Mrs ___, my name is Dr _____. Is it OK if I ask you a few questions?"

Look at her. Is she dressed appropriately? Is she agitated?

"How are you feeling?

How long have you been feeling like this, since the baby was born?

Do you feel tired most of the time?

Do you feel hopeless?

Are you coping with your baby?

Are you crying a lot?

Have you lost interest in life?

How is your appetite?

How is sleep?

Do you feel like harming yourself/your baby?

Do you think someone else is trying to harm your baby?

Are you hearing or seeing things when they are not there?"

About pregnancy

"Is this your first baby?
Was the pregnancy normal?
What was your delivery like?
How was your mood during pregnancy?
Any history of depression?
Any support at home?
Any problems at home?"

Tell patient

"Baby blues is very common. It affects 1 in 2 women. It usually starts in the first 3–4 days. It disappears itself and what you need is rest, good diet and lots of support from your family. The children's doctor has seen little ____ and he is completely normal, so enjoy him!"

On the other hand

"Post-natal depression is less common but more serious; affects 5%. Psychosis is even rarer (0.3%). Post-natal depression usually occurs between 1 and 6 months. They usually require medical treatment. If frank psychosis, then admit as an emergency to Mother-Baby-Unit.

AMMENORHOEA FOR A LENGTH OF TIME

Possible scenario is someone who is mid-aged with irregular, infrequent periods or someone who is around 50 having sweats, etc.

Questions to ask

- Menarche
- LMP
- Periods regular before – cycle length/pattern
- Contraception used, e.g. been on depot? Any chance you could be pregnant?
- Pregnancies? Breastfeeding?
- Any bleeding after pregnancies (Sheehans)?
- Any surgical terminations (Ashermans)?
- Feeling tired/ weight gain/loss of hair (hypo-thyroidism)?
- How is your mood? In stress?
- Increased hair growth/acne (polycystic ovarian dis.)?
- Any hot sweats/mood changes?
- Any milk discharge from breasts/any headaches (prolactinonomas)?
- Any weightloss?

HYPEREMESIS

Main aspects

- If ketones in urine, admit for i.v. fluids and antiemetic.
- Check urine for ketones at least twice a day.
- Most antiemetics are safe in pregnancy.
- Scan to look for twins/molar pregnancy.

CERVICAL SMEAR RESULTS

Screening Programme in UK

- Start after 20th birthday.
- Every 3–5 years until 65 yrs old (some places recall every 3 yrs, others every 5 yrs).

RESULTS	ACTION
NEGATIVE INADEQUATE	Recall at 3–5 yrs repeat in 3 months. After two consecutive inadequate smears send for colposcopy
BORDERLINE	Repeat in 3 months. If three borderlines then need colposcopy.
MILD DYSKARYOSIS (CIN 1)	Repeat in 6 months. If get a second dyskaryosis then for colposcopy
MODERATE/SEVERE DYSKARYOSIS (CIN 2/3)	Colposcopy
SUSPECTED CANCER	Colposcopy

SPECULUM AND VAGINAL EXAMINATION (BIMANUAL)

If asked to do smear then you'll be doing a speculum as well. Generally you do a speculum first and them pv. If examiner says 'examine this lady's pelvic organs', then you need to do both speculum and pv. If only asked to do bimanual then say to examiner "I would generally start with speculum first" but you don't need to do it as not asked. The examiner will probably ask you to just carry on with smear. If doing smear, always explain to the patient that it is a screening test to detect abnormal cells that may move onto being cancer.

1. Introduce yourself to the patient and explain that due to the nature of her problem you have to examine her down below. This will entail a speculum examination like when she had a smear. If she have never had a smear then tell her that you shall have to insert a speculum down below so that you could see the cervix and vaginal properly. It is uncomfortable but not painful. You shall then have to do an internal. This will entail inserting your finger down below into the vagina so that you can assess the size and position of the womb. Also, you will able to check for any abnormality. You will have chaperone and ensure privacy. Lock any doors.

2. Ask patient if she wants to go to the toilet. Ask her to undress from waist downwards

and give a blanket to cover herself. You shall wait outside while she is undressing.

3. Wear gloves and start with inspection of the vulva. Look for ulcers, warts, discharge, swelling, cysts, scars, etc.

4. Ask the patient to bear down – look for any prolapse. Ask her to cough – look for stress incontinence. Ask her to lie with ankles together and knees apart for speculum examination.

5. Tell the patient that you shall be inserting the speculum. It may feel cold and feel uncomfortable. Should not be painful – "If it hurts, please tell me." Check speculum that it works and put lubrication on (KY jelly) – this is very important. Don't forget it! Spread the labia apart gently with left hand. Insert speculum in sideways first pushing downward and posterior. Once you have inserted the speculum about 1 inch turn in round to the correct position. Once fully in, dilate speculum and lock position.

6. Once you have found the cervix, look for any masses, ectropion, bleeding, etc.

7. Take triple swabs – endocervical (gonnorheoea, chlamydia) and high vaginal (bacterial vaginosis, thrush, etc.). [NB: the gonnorhoea and HVS (high vaginal swab) is the black one. The chlamydia one is pink.]

8. Take smear if indicated. Use either an Ayre's spatula (wooden) or the plastic brush. To get smear insert the pointed bit or bristles of brush into the cervical os and turn clockwise

360°. Immediately fix the cells onto the slide. This is done by brushing along the slide twice. Fix it with fixator (e.g. cytofix) straight away. (NB: the slide should be labelled with the patient's detail in pencil already by your assistant or you do it at the start.)

9. Loosen screws and remove speculum gently. Close blades fully before removing speculum.

10. Then tell patient that you want to do an internal examination like mentioned before. Put KY jelly on your index and middle finger. No need to change gloves from before. Insert your index finger only into the vagina. Assess for any masses, polyps, etc. in vagina. Assess cervical excitation (get in ectopic and PID). Insert two fingers (index and mid) and feel cervix and try and push uterus up. Your left hand should be on the abdomen to feel the uterus (bimanual examination). Feel for size of uterus (describe it in terms of weeks in pregnancy or in terms of comparison to fruits, e.g. size of a plum). Explain if retroverted or anterverted (anterverted moves easier). Is it mobile/hard?

   While still doing pv examination, move your left hand into the adnexa. You should move your fingers into the lateral fornices. Feel for any masses or tenderness.

11. Thank patient and ask her to get dressed.

NB: Always do speculum first and then the bimanual. This is because by doing bimanual first you will be introducing germs so your swabs will not be accurate.

Do not take smear if on period as the result will come back unsatisfactory.

Explain the results of the smear will take a couple of weeks. If abnormal, you will contact her directly but she is welcome to ring up for results.

BREAST EXAMINATION

You will be given a dummy breast and asked to examine the breast. Make sure you talk through the examination and get consent. ALWAYS ASK FOR A CHAPERONE. Explain to the patient that "due to the nature of your problem I have to examine your breasts. Is that OK? I have got a nurse to act as a chaperone. I will have to start by looking."

1. **Expose** the whole of upper half of patient and ask patient to sit at 45°.

2. **Look** at breasts for symmetry, contour, size. Look at the skin for any puckering, 'peau d'orange', ulcers, lumps, etc.

3. Look at nipples for any discharge, retraction/inversion. Any extra nipples? – (quite common)

4. Ask patient to put arms behind head and look for any changes. Look at back of breasts.

5. Ask patient to place hands on hips – this relaxes pectoral muscles and makes lumps more obvious.

6. **Palpate** – feel with flat of fingers. Go round as if a circle moving inwards from the outside. Any lumps? – position, tenderness, temperature, shape, size, surface, edge, etc.

7. Is lump fixed to skin or is it tethered (attached to the subcutaneous fibres and this causes skin tethering).

8. Is lump fixed to muscle – feel mobility of lump first when patient is relaxing with arms

on hips. Then feel when hands pushed against hips thus contracted pectoral muscles. If attached to muscle then mobility is less when the muscle is contracted.

9. Palplate nipple – if any discharge, take swab.
10. Feel axilla and supraclavicular region for any **lymph nodes**.
11. Examine arms for any oedema.
12. Tell the examiner "I would like to examine the abdomen to check for presence of any ascites/hepatomegaly."

NB: Current breast screening programme: single oblique mammography every 3 yrs between 50 and 64 yrs.

PAEDIATRICS

PAEDIATRIC CASES

Possible scenarios

- Mother thinks child has meningitis – reassure
- Child has symptoms of DM – take history
- Diarrhoea and vomiting – telephone advise
- A child is born stillborn – speak to family
- Child has asthma – explain implications
- Febrile convulsion
- Nocturnal enuresis

TALKING TO MOTHER ON PHONE

A child has a temperature and some throat and ear pain. Being irritable. Mother is on the phone.

(NB: In telephone OSCEs you will be given a telephone and the examiner will be sitting behind the screen acting as the patient. Don't panic – stay cool. It's probably easier as no one is watching!)

"Hello, how are you. It's Dr _____. Can you just confirm who I am speaking to?

"Mrs Jones. Hello Doc."

"What can I do for you Mrs Jones?"

"Well it's John. He's ever so ill. He's got a temperature and been pulling at his left ear. He has not slept at all last night."

"Have you given him anything for it?"

"Calpol. But it's no good."

"Has he been playing and eating?"

"No, he's in bed."

"I think you should bring John to the surgery. We need to have a good look at his ears and throat. He may have an infection for which he needs antibiotics. Also, his temperature is not coming down so we can give him ibuprofen. Do you have any other questions. Do you understand? If you cannot get to the surgery we can come out to see you."

Here it is important you ask questions about how child is and what mum has done already. More important is that you get mum to bring child in. Don't panic mum!

?MENINGITIS

A mother thinks her child has meningitis. Reassure her that it is only an ear infection.

"Hello, Mrs Jones; I am Dr ____. How could I help you?

"Paul, is very unwell. The other doctor said he has an ear infection but I think it is more serious."

"What are you worried about?"

"Meningitis"

"Well, Mrs Jones. Looking at Paul he seems to have a temperature. His temperature is up at 37.8° but with meningitis it goes much higher. Also, looking at his ears there seems to be signs of an infection. For this you have been given antibiotics.

Also, in meningitis the child is drowsy and has a severe headache. A child can be irritable even after a viral infection and irritability does not necessarily mean meningitis. Do you understand?"

"Yes Dr"

"Is John sleeping all the time or does the light bother him?"

"No, he seems to be playing."

"Is he eating or drinking?"

"Bits and pieces."

"I am certain he does not have meningitis. However, I understand your concern. If John's temperature does not come down or you think he is getting worse, bring him to the surgery or hospital. If you notice a rash which does not disappear on pressing a see-through glass over it – then straight to hospital. Do you understand? If at any point you are concerned just ring us or come to the surgery. If you are unhappy with this chat you can bring John to the surgery."

(NB: If mum is unhappy with the child, ask her to come in.)

"Thank you."

ADVISE ABOUT DIRRHOEA

Mother is on the phone asking about child who has diarrhoea.

"Hello, Mrs Jones. It's Dr ＿＿＿ here. How can I help?

"It's Bob, he's had diarrhoea since yesterday."

"OK Mrs Jones. May I ask a few questions?"

"Yes"

"How long has it been like that?

How many times is he going per day?

Any blood/mucus/pus?

Is it watery or just formed stools but more often?

Is he complaining of tummy pain?

Have you been on holiday recently?

Anyone else affected?

Is his tongue dry?

How many times is he passing water (<3 = dehydrated)

Is he playing about or is he sleeping all the time?

Is he vomiting too?"

(If you think he may be dehydrated, i.e. less, urine, quiet, not playing – admit, if on the other hand child seems well then advise oral rehydration, e.g. diarolyte or make up own rehydration fluid – boil 2 pints water and let it cool, add 10 teaspoons of sugar and 1 teaspoon of salt.)

NB: It is always best to ask mum to bring child to surgery so that you can see for yourself. Or offer to visit at home.

STILLBORN BABY

Couple have had stillborn baby – talk to them

(Also, read 'Breaking Bad News')

"Hello, my name is Dr ____. Is it OK if I talk to you about what has happened?"

"I understand that it is very difficult for you and am sorry about what has happened. However, it is important that you understand that it is something that can happen commonly.

It is possible for you to see your baby, take a photograph, footprint or lock of hair. You can organise for a private funeral or we can make arrangements for this.

As there may be a reason why this has happened to your baby, it is important we look for any possible causes. By this we may be able to prevent this in future. We would like to take some blood from the baby and yourselves. If we examine the baby thoroughly by doing a postmortem, it may give us more clues. However, this is not compulsory and we shall let you decide if you are unhappy about a post-mortem.

At the postmortem, a specialist doctor will look at the baby's organs. Everything will be put back as it was and nothing will be removed. If you are not happy about a postmortem we can just take a small sample of tissue from the baby.

As you may produce breast milk, we can give you tablets to stop this. You shall have to take the tablet for around two weeks.

We shall give you a certificate of stillbirth which you need to take to the Registrar's office within 42 days.

There are some societies that can provide more information: one of these is SANDS, we can give you their number and also the contact number for the bereavement counsellor if you like.

With regard to getting pregnant again, it is advisable to wait another 6 months to 1 year.

We would like to see you in 6 weeks time to discuss your blood results and plans for future pregnancy."

COLIC

Child has colic—talk to mother

Colic is common and distressing. However, it does not harm the baby, and it usually goes by the age of 3–4 months.

A healthy new-born baby may have periods of crying, typically in the early evening. For no apparent reason they cry as if in pain. The usual methods of comforting do not seem to work very well. They don't want to feed, they may pull their knees up, and sometimes their abdomen (tummy) appears to 'rumble'.

The rest of the time the baby is fine. However, the bouts of colic occur regularly, usually every evening. Bouts of colic gradually become less frequent, and have gone in most babies by the age of 3–4 months. Colic does not harm the baby, and there are no long-term problems once the colic goes.

The cause of colic is not known. There are many theories. There is some evidence that sensitivity to cow's milk may sometimes play a part. There is no test for colic, and there is nothing abnormal found if a doctor examines the baby.

There is no treatment that cures colic. Parents have their own way of coping and may find different things helpful. Try not to despair. Colic has usually gone by 3–4 months of age, often much sooner. Sometimes parents become angry, tearful, or resentful towards a baby with colic. These are normal and common emotions. The following may help.

Even new-born babies may sense anxiety. This can make things worse. Try to create a relaxed atmosphere. If possible, have a rest and meal before the colic begins (usually in the evening). The more rested and relaxed you are, the better you will be able to cope.

It is natural to try and soothe a crying baby. However, there is some evidence to suggest that 'over handling' of crying babies may make things worse. It is acceptable to leave a baby to cry for short periods if you are satisfied he/she is not hungry, wet, or ill. Try not to immediately pick the baby up as soon he/she starts crying. Try to avoid holding the baby for long periods. This may be difficult as the natural instinct is to try to comfort. However, a colicky baby may simply not be comforted. Leaving the baby in the cot for a short while may be the best thing to do at times.

A sensitivity to cow's milk is one theory for colic. Some babies cry less if cow's milk is stopped. This does not occur in most babies. However, it may be worth trying without cow's milk for one week. If the baby is breast fed, this means mum having no dairy products as part of the cow's milk can get into breast milk. If the baby is bottle fed, this means changing to a 'hypoallergenic' feed. A pharmacist will be able to advise on a suitable milk powder.

If there is an improvement, then continue without cow's milk until the baby is three months old. It is not a true 'allergy', and after colic has settled the baby will be able to take cow's milk again. If there is no improvement after one week, there is no point continuing without cow's milk and you should resume normal milk feeds.

Friends or other family members may be willing to help. Try and avoid several people fussing at once as this may cause anxiety. It may be sensible to leave the coping to one person at a time. Take it in turns if you have help. If possible, it is good to have 'time-out' and leave someone else to look after the baby for a few hours.

Gripe water, Infacol, etc. have been popular in the past. There is little evidence that they have any effect to relieve colic.

Some foods can get into breast milk. It is difficult to prove if colic is made worse by foods eaten by the mother. Some women say that their baby's colic becomes worse if they eat garlic or spices. Some women have said that stopping caffeine improves the situation. Caffeine is found in tea, coffee, and cola. It is also added to some painkillers such as Solpadeine. If you suspect a food, drink, or medicine is making colic worse, try going without it for a week. It is unlikely to be a cause of colic if there is no improvement within a week.

Some people say that 'white noise' helps to soothe colicky babies. White noise is background, non-specific noise such as made by vacuum cleaners, washing machines, etc. You can even buy tapes of white noise which claim to soothe crying babies. Again, there is lack of proof that this is effective in most babies.

Crying babies may settle on car journeys. It is possibly the white noise of the car engine and the gentle movements of the car that do the trick.

CRYING BABY

Crying all night

Here you need to make sure both mother and child do not have a problem.

Questions for baby
- "How long has it been going on for?
- Does he sleep at all? For how long?
- What about during the day?
- Feeding problems?
- Does he draw legs up when crying (colic)?
- Stool and waterworks fine?
- Fever?
- Where does he sleep?
- Recent immunisations?"

Question for mother
- "Any other children?
- How was pregnancy/delivery/postnatal period?
- Any helpers at home?
- How is your mood?
- Any thoughts about harming yourself/your baby?
- How is your mood?"

You have to come to a conclusion, i.e. does baby have a cold/ colic, etc. or is it the mother that is not coping.

POLYDIPSIA

Child with polydipsia — Take history from mum

Questions
- "How old is your child?
- How long he/she had the problem?
- How many times does he pass water?
- Any problem with stools?
- Any weight-loss?
- How is appetite?
- Any fever?
- Complaining of burning on passing water or tummy pain?
- Is she always complaining of being thirsty?
- Any family history of diabetes?"

Explain to mother: "Your child has been passing a lot of urine and also loosing weight. I think she may have diabetes. However, there is also a possibility that it may be an infection. Either way we need to admit your child and do some tests. Even if it is an infection, we will need to treat it and follow your child regularly.

Diabetes can be easily treated by giving insulin. You child will be kept in hospital while you and your child learn about diabetes and how to treat it. We will refer you to specialist who will advise."

ASTHMA

Child is diagnosed with asthma – talk to mother

Introduce, etc.

"Hello. Is it OK if I talk to you about asthma which little John has?"

"Asthma is very common nowadays. We do not know exactly why this is. Whether it is because of pollution or if we are getting better at diagnosing it.

In asthma the airways are hypersensitive to some things such as dust. Things like dust will cause the airways to narrow making the wheeze and cough. Treatment is possible with inhaler. We will teach you and child how to use these. If asthma is not controlled with just one inhaler we can give another. You may have heard that we also use a steroid inhaler. It is important that you know that the dose of steroid is minimal and will not affect the growth of your child.

If at any point you think that asthma is getting worse, then you need to see a doctor.

John can go to school and holidays as normal. He can also play sports normally. It may be advisable to take his inhaler with sports if activity makes his breathing worse.

Let his teachers know he has asthma.

There are some things you can do help his asthma at home. Cats and dogs make it worse, also keeping the carpet clean helps. Avoid using fluffy bed linen and pillows.

When children have asthma they sometimes also have eczema or hay fever. We can treat these effectively too.

It is important that you understand that asthma can be easily controlled if treatment is taken regularly. Also, many children grow out of asthma."

Some questions to ask in history

- How is his breathing affected?
- Any cough – worse at night?
- Any pets?
- Is sleep affected?
- Is school affected?
- Any eczema, hay fever?
- Any FH of asthma, etc.
- What treatment are you on? Do you take it regularly?
- Check inhaler technique
- What is normal PFR?
- Any admissions for asthma?
- Any ICU admissions?

FEBRILE CONVULSION

A child has had a febrile convulsion – talk to parent.

"Hello, my name is Dr ____. Is it OK if I talk about John with you?"

"As you are aware he had a fit at home today. This must have been very scary to you. Let me reassure you that it was because he had a high temperature. It does not mean he has epilepsy and neither does it mean that he will grow up to have epilepsy.

He had something called a 'febrile convulsion'. This is a fit due to raised temperature. The temperature was probably up due to an infection.

Febrile convulsions are very common. They occur in 3% of children and are usually between the ages 6 month and 3 yrs. As your child has had a convulsion there is a chance that in future if John's temperature is too high it may happen again.

If John's temperature is high in future then you need to bring it down with paracetamol and ibuprofen. Also, use tepid sponging. The best way to prevent a convulsion is to keep the temperature down.

However, if he does have a fit again then you should leave him alone. Try not to move him around or hold him. Once he stops, put him in the recovery position. If the fit last more than 5 minutes call the ambulance."

NB: Any child with first febrile convulsion needs to be admitted. For the second one it is not necessary.

NOCTURNAL ENURESIS

- Very common: 15% of 5 yr olds and 3% of 10 yr olds.
- Genetic delay in acquiring sphincter competence.
- Boys:Girls = 2:1
- Most children with nocturnal enuresis are psychologically normal.
- Rule out – DM, UTI, constipation.
- Treatment – star chart, bell + pad, desmopressin spray.

NON-ACCIDENTAL INJURY

This is a difficult station. The scenario may be that you have seen a child in A&E and suspect NAI. Talk to the mother.

Important things in history

- Several injuries
- Delayed presentation
- Various ages of injuries
- Injury does not match history given
- Parents seem distant from child
- Child withdrawn
- Frequent attendees
- Failure to thrive
- Unexplained floppiness
- Signs of neglect

WHAT DO YOU SAY TO PARENTS

Tell examiner that before you speak to the parents you would like to speak to your seniors, get paediatric advise and check if the child is on the 'Child Protection Register' (this is a register of all the children in that area at risk).

Tell mother/father

"Hello, my name is Dr _____ and I have been looking after John. From our examinations and tests I think we need to admit John for more investigations. We also need to observe him and get advise from the children's specialists. I do not think there is anything serious going on but observation will help with the diagnosis."

If parents are getting aggressive, you would get your senior (registrar or consultant) to speak to them. If family disappear from the department then you would speak to seniors and paediatricians and find out if there are any people, e.g. social services, you need to alert.

PSYCHIATRY

TAKING A PSYCHIATRIC HISTORY

Before you even start LOOK:

- Eye contact
- Are they appropriately dressed
- Movements are they showing excessive movements – agitated

History

PC: What are the symptoms

Effect on work, life, sex, etc.

Appetite

Family History: Ask about parents and siblings. Age and any illnesses. How do they get on?

Personal History: Split this into groups chronologically, i.e.:

- Childhood: stable family?
- School: finish school? Any qualifications?
- Sexual Hx: menarch, sexually active?
- Marriage: separations, relationships,
- Children
- Occupation

- Forensic: been in trouble with law
- Present social circumstances: accommodation, etc.

Pre-Morbid Personalities: say "Mr Jones, I'd like to ask you some questions about what sort of person you were before you became ill". Ask about interests, mood, habits, including alcohol.

NB: It is unlikely you'd be asked to do the above. You only have 5 minutes and will probably only get given one psychiatry case. More likely you will get something like an elderly confused man, suicide assessment or history from someone who is depressed.

MENTAL STATE EXAMINATION

You may be asked to do this: Given a scenario where some young chap has come is confused and is having hallucinations. NB: You only have 5 minutes in the exam so I have summarised the important things.

Say to patient: "Hello, my name is Dr _____. I would like to have a chat with you about yourself. Is that OK?"

Appearance and Behaviour

Conscious level
Is patient appropriately dressed?
Any agitated movements?
Is he aggressive to the interviewer?

Speech

Is it too fast?
Does speech follow a logical pattern?
'Flight of ideas'?

Mood

Ask: "How have you been feeling recently?
Are you feeling hopeless?
As if life isn't worth living?"
If he says "yes" to this, then ask questions regarding SUICIDE

Thoughts

Suicidal ideas: "Have you ever thought of harming
   yourself?

Have you planned how you would do it?

Do you intend to carry it out?"

Any delusions (a delusion is a false belief held
with conviction, i.e. patient is certain it is true even
though others tell it isn't, for example, someone is
feeling as if neighbours are going to kill him as he is
evil)?

Do you think somebody wants to harm you?

Do you think somebody is controlling you?

Do you think somebody is controlling your thoughts,
removing your thoughts or that your thoughts are
getting known by everybody?" (broadcasting)

Perception

Any hallucinations : "Do you ever hear voices when
   no one else is there?

What do they say?

Are they your own thoughts inside your head, or of
   someone else?"

Any visual hallucination: "Have you been seeing
   anything unusual?"

Orientation

Say "I would like to ask you questions to find out if
   you are keeping up to date with things:

Day – Date-Year-Name of place we are in,

Person – 'who am I'?"

Attention and Concentration

"Now we will do a bit of maths to check your concentration:

'Minus sevens from a hundred'?"

Registration and Short-term Memory

"I will say a few names and I would like you to repeat them after me (books, pens, doors, cars, etc...)"

"What you have eaten this breakfast?

Do you remember the name of UK's Prime Minister during 1980s?

When World War II started and finished?"

Remote Memory

"Who is the prime-minister at present?

What date was it when you got married?"

Insight

"Do you think you have an illness?

Do you know what might have caused it?

Do you need help?"

** In the end, summarise your findings and talk through it in sections, i.e.

'The patient is not appropriately dressed for a hot day and seems agitated. His speech is fast and does not make sense. His mood seems to be low and he is showing features of suicidal intent. I would like to admit him for this. He is having some delusions in the sense that he feels his neighbour is out to kill him......'

MINI MENTAL STATE EXAMINATION

Scenario could be some elderly fellow found wandering on the road. Brought back by the police. Your aim would be to assess mental function and more importantly compare this to his normal mental state, i.e. is this acute confusional state or dementia? Causes, e.g. infection, subdural, etc.

The best is to read the *Oxford Handbook of Clinical Medicine,* pp. 76-77.

Or split into:

Orientation

1. What is the

  Year

  Season

  Date

  Day

  Month

2. Where are we?

  State

  County

  Town/City

  Hospital

  Floor

Registration

   3. Name three objects, i.e. ask the patient to say all three after you have said them. One point for each correct answer. Ask him/her to remember these for later.

Attention and Calculation

   4. Serial sevens (i.e. 100 minus 7). Stop after five correct answers. One point for each correct answer.

      Alternative is to spell WORLD backwards.

Recall

   5. Ask name of the three objects told in 3. One point for each correct answer.

Language

   6. Point to watch and pencil. Ask patient to name. One point for each correct answer – 3 points.

   7. Ask patient to repeat 'no ifs, ands, or buts' – 1 point.

   8. Follow a three-stage command, e.g. "take paper in your hand. Fold the paper. Put it on the floor now."

   9. Make patient read and obey the following: "CLOSE YOUR EYES"

  10. Ask patient to write a sentence (should contain subject and an object and also make sense)

  11. Draw the two hexagons jointed.

= Total 30

Another quick way is
THE NEWCASTLE SCALE

1. Age (nearest yr)	1 point
2. Time (nearest hr)	1 point
3. Address to be repeated at end, e.g. "Can you remember this address "10 Rose Cottage' – I will ask you to repeat it at the end."	1 point
4. Year	1 point
5. Name of place we are in	1 point
6. Recognition of person, e.g. "Who is this with you?"	1 point
7. D.O.B.	1 point
8. When was World War 2?	1 point
9. Who is the queen?	1 point
10. Count back from 20-1	1 point

Repeat that address from '3'

This would quickly assess orientation, short-term memory, and attention. Score of less than 8 = cognitive impairment.

I would suggest you do this for the exam as it checks for acute confusion. These are the situations you will get in the exam. Also, you cannot possibly do the other 30 point test in 5 minutes; the 30 score is more for dementia, etc.

ALCOHOL

Possible scenarios

- **Patient admitted with alcohol intoxication — take a history**

- **You find raised MCV on routine pre-op bloods tests – take alcohol history**

- **Patient has gout – you suspect increased alcohol intake**

You should never be judgemental and always treat alcoholism as a disease. It has both medical and social implications. You have to mention these in your discussion with the patient.

Screening

Questions to ask

CAGE	
C	Do you feel you have to CUT down on your drinking?
A	Do you get ANNOYED with people telling you how much you drink?
G	Do you feel GUILTY about your drinking?
E	Do you feel drink in the morning (EYE OPENER)?

* If the patient has two or more then has alcohol problem.

Another good one is CONTROL.

- Can you always **C**ontrol your drinking?
- Has alcohol ever led you to **N**eglect your family or work?
- What **T**ime do you start drinking?
- Do friends comment on how much you drink or ask you to **R**educe?
- Do you drink in the morning to **O**vercome a hangover?
- Go through average day alcohol, **L**eaving nothing out.

Other important things to ask about:

- Who do you drink with? Do you drink alone?
- What job do you do?
- Take any other drugs?
- Ever been in trouble with law for drinking?
- How is your health otherwise?
- Have you tried to cut down in past?
- Any family history of addiction?

Once you have diagnosed alcoholism, you have to counsel the patient regarding this. Things to say:

- "Sir, after speaking to you and looking at your blood results, I think you drink too much, do you agree?
- Do you know that alcohol has serious effects on your health. These can be in the short term such as accidents, aspiration pneumonia, social problems. Also, will cause problems in the

future if you carry on like this such as liver failure, brain damage (Korsakoffs), bursting of blood vessels in your food pipe and heart disease.

- Do you understand?

- There are a few things we can do to help such as give you contact details of the alcohol-team and also numbers for Alcohol Anonymous, etc. There are also a few tablets available to help you reduce alcohol" (antabuse, vitamins for malnutrition, etc.)

DRUG ABUSE

Possible scenario could be

- Young person comes in with DVT secondary to i.v. drug use.
- Someone with side-effects of morphine withdrawal (runny nose, yawning, irritable, sleep affected).
- Someone coming to see you who wants to come off heroine.

Questions to ask

- What do you take? (list)
- How much?
- How do you take it, e.g. intravenous, sniff, etc.?
- How do you pay for it? (prostitution, stealing)
- Been in trouble with law for it?
- How long been taking?
- Why started?
- Any withdrawal symptoms?
- Dependence?
- Alcohol problem?

Counselling the patient should involve talking about what she takes and why.

How you can help, e.g. by referring to the drugs team in the community.

Tell the patient about the risks of taking drugs:

- Infections (e.g. hepatitis and HIV from i.v. use)

- DVT/PE
- High doses of opioids leading to slowing/stopping breathing
- Social and criminal problems
- If prostitution, then risk of STD
- Dependence and cravings

NB: overdoses of opioids you treat with narcan (naloxone 400–800 mcg)

If someone comes to see you wanting to come off heroin, etc. you would again take the history as above. Finding out what he/she takes, how and where does the finance come from. The mainstay for opioids is something called METHADONE. A liquid drug which is given instead of heroin. The most important thing is that the patient has to be committed to stopping heroin. The doctor has to see the patient regularly so that he can wean off the methadone too. Also, there are important aspects like whether this patient is selling the methadone?

NB: If asked to write a prescription for a controlled drug, you have to write as follows:

'Please dispense Methadone 20 mg (twenty milligrams). Provide one hundred millilitres please.'

The numbers have to be written in words. Also, you have to write down the full name and address of the patient.

PARACETAMOL OR OTHER DRUG OVERDOSE

Paracetamol

Paracetamol is one of the most common overdose drugs, probably because it is so easily available. The British National Formulary and OHCM (p. 796) have some good guidelines.

Basically, you have to be able to recognise and interpret the graph (see below). The main points are:

- Check levels once 4 hours since ingestion.
- If overdose is staggered (i.e. multiple overdoses over some time), then treat as levels could be misleading.
- Treatment is with N-acetylcysteine i.v. (doses in BNF/OHCM – you don't need to know).
- On the graph there is a 'high risk treatment line' which is for those people also taking enzyme-inducing drugs (carbamezepine, phenytoin, rifampicin, alcohol, etc.)
- If signs of liver failure, send to specialist liver unit straight away.
- Bloods tests to do: toxic screen (measure paracetamol and salicylates level), FBC, UEs, clotting, LFTs.

NB: With any overdose you have to do a full PSYCHIATRIC ASSESMENT and get the on-call psychiatrist to do this too. ADMIT PATIENT.

Other possible overdose drugs are TRICYCLICS – these can cause serious cardiac dysrthymias, so always do ECG. If abnormal ECG treatment is sodium bicarbonate. They can also depress GCS so may need ICU.

- Gastric lavage is no longer used in this country. May be in exceptional cases it might still be. Charcoal – give if patient presents within 1 hr of overdose.

- Remember you can always check out TOXBASE (gives information on overdoses/poisons) and there is also the specialist POISON CENTRES, e.g. Guys Poison Centre.

* See Paracetamol Poisoning Graph in Booklet or Course

DEPRESSION

Possible scenarios

- **Someone has been diagnosed with cancer and is feeling low. Take history.**
- **Insomnia**
- **Weightloss**
- **Someone is trying to commit suicide**

Taking a history from someone who is depressed:

Important questions to ask

- Non-verbal: How is she dressed? All black? Eye contact? Crying? Posture?
- Is there loss of interest in life? (anhedonia)
- How is appetite? (weightloss but can be weight gain)
- Are you waking up early?
- Is mood worse in mornings? (in depression it is)
- Reduced sex drive: "How often are you having intercourse?"
- Reduced concentration: "What is your concentration like?"
- Feeling worthless, guilty: "Have you been feeling useless?"
- Thoughts of death/suicide: "Have you thought about ending it all?"
- Palpitations, exacerbation of asthma, etc.
- PMH